To Brenda —

The New
E.A.T.
and Be Healthy

*for your health
and happy life!*

Judy Fields

Judy Fields, MHS, RD, FADA

ISBN: 0-9631434-4-1
ISBN-13: 9780963143440
Library of Congress Control Number: 2011943662
CreateSpace Independent Publishing Platform
North Charleston, South Carolina

DEDICATION

The book is dedicated to the memory of my mother, Lucille J. Coontz, who provided the 'seed' money for the first edition. I also acknowledge the thousands of patients I have counseled over the past years. I have learned from each of them and worked to coach them in the process of not only losing weight, but mastering maintenance.

ACKNOWLEDGMENTS

I would like to thank the following for their help in making the *New E.A.T. and Be Healthy* a reality:

Daisy Lindner-Stoutsenberger, R.N., and the late Peter G. Lindner, M.D., my mentors, who have guided me in my approach to weight loss counseling.

Priscilla McCrea, dietetic intern and now Registered Dietitian, who assisted with reviewing the revised manuscript.

Kellie Slingerland, artist and client, who graciously illustrated the weight resistant exercises, and who has lost a total of 115 lb. to date. This is no small feat, especially considering she started in the seventh grade and is now finishing high school and pursuing her dream of a culinary arts degree.

James W. Fields, my best friend and loving husband, who has inspired, supported and encouraged me to pursue my dream.

Chapter 1

Introduction

The Perspective of a Successful Loser –Steve

When I was a child, food was used as a reward in my home. It was also used for comfort, for sympathy, and for all celebrations. In fact, food was the focal point of all that seemed to be "good" in my life. In addition to this belief, I inherited a family disposition towards gaining fat easily. When I reached nine years of age, I was quite husky, even though I was a typically active kid.

When I was twelve years old, my family went into the bakery business. We all worked long hours at the bakery, but the "good" part (at least in my eyes) was that we could eat anything we wanted. Lots of choices were readily available and everything we made was really good. Throughout my high school years, I think I probably had only a couple of good meals per week; everything else was fast food or a hastily made sandwich in the bakery.

I married young, and my new bride and I began our home. In the early years of our marriage, we prepared whatever foods tasted the best to us. Good nutrition, or even the thought of what might be best for us to eat, never entered into our meal planning. Taste, convenience, and quantity were the only factors that mattered. After our children arrived, my wife tried to fix healthier foods. As our little family grew, I went into the shoe business. Not only was this a sedentary job, but I also spent a lot of time alone and did a lot of snacking—all high-carbohydrate, high-fat choices. My weight began to climb, rising to 240 pounds.

Periodically I did make an effort to lose weight, trying different weight loss plans. I enjoyed Weight Watchers, losing thirty-five to forty pounds on their eating program. Unfortunately, after I left the weekly program, I regained the weight back over the next year. But it did cause me to develop an interest in vegetables and in watching my portions of meat.

When my marriage ended some time later, I lost fifty pounds in less than six months without trying. This, however, is certainly not a happy way to reduce. My weight seemed to settle right around two hundred pounds, and I became more active just trying to occupy my time. In addition to my full-time job, I began to work two part-time jobs-- one in an emergency room and one as an ambulance tech. I never averaged more than four hours of sleep a night, and I rarely ate a balanced meal. In fact, my "meals" were mostly greasy fast food and lots of alcohol.

Now in my mid-thirties and alone, I began to travel even more for the shoe company employing me. I often stayed on the road for up to six weeks at a time. Having an expense account, I ate all my meals in restaurants and bars, washing rich meals down with ten to twelve alcoholic drinks per day. After some eight years of this lifestyle, my weight rose to 320 pounds. I began to hate myself as I felt steadily worse physically. I was smoking up to four packs of cigarettes a day, and my "exercise" consisted of walking from airplanes to baggage claims to rental cars.

About this time, my mother died of cancer, and I began to think about my own mortality. After an unpleasant assessment of my life, such as it was, I decided I'd better make some changes—fast. I decided that the first change would be to stop drinking. I will always remember one night on the road in Idaho Falls, Idaho, where I had met a fellow in the bar before dinner, as the beginning of a turning point in my life. The two of us spent nearly two hours drinking, and I consumed ten double Staley's on the rocks (thirty ounces of alcohol!). After dinner, I made some calls before going to bed and got up the next morning as if nothing unusual had happened the night before. This really shook me up when I stopped to think of my body being so alcohol soaked that thirty ounces of booze in a two-hour period had such little effect on my physical state.

I began to let myself remember some of the tragic results of drinking that I was exposed to when I worked in the emergency room. I knew it was time to stop the cycle, and I made my decision. As I became more and more determined to stop my out-of-control drinking, a growing feeling came over me that this would give me control of one corner of my life. This was the beginning of a sense of personal empowerment. It felt good to know that I could stand my ground when others tried to get me to join them for drinks.

Six months later, I realized that I was actually in pretty bad shape, in spite of cutting out alcohol. I decided to get a complete physical check-up and the news was not good. My blood pressure was up to 160/100 in spite of multiple medications I was already taking. The doctor said I definitely needed to lose weight, stop smoking and cut out all caffeine. I took my prescriptions, stayed off alcohol and contemplated which impossible mountain I would try to scale first. My life seemed to be just one mountain after another—a whole range of them, in fact!

The first mountainous goal the doctor convinced me to set was to stop smoking. Afraid of failing, I refused to even try, and I ignored his warnings. I had always had a love/hate relationship with smoking. I loved the feeling it gave me and I hated it for the control it held over my life. I used a well-known nicotine gum to help my cravings and managed to stop smoking and get off caffeine at the same time. I'm still amazed by this, for it was the hardest thing I think I have ever done. Nicotine is a powerful addiction, one that I have to fight minute to minute. But I have never had another cigarette.

My weight, though, continued to climb, finally reaching a high of 360 pounds. Self-hatred began to churn inside of me again. My weight was now physically impacting every area of my life. Whenever I went to a store, I had to drive around the parking lot (sometimes more than once) to find a space close to the doors, as it was difficult for me to walk any distance. Airplane seats became almost impossible. Clothes had become very hard for me to find. I felt powerless to do anything.

Food was my enemy, and yet I was forced into repeated encounters with this enemy every day of my life. All addictions are very hard to overcome, but food is a doubly hard addiction to deal with, as you cannot walk away and just cut it out of your life. Many well-meaning people were trying to get me to do something for my health's sake, but this only made me more depressed. To compensate for the depression, I just ate more. During this valley of my life, I moved to Sacramento, California.

About this time, I began to have trouble reading and was forced to admit that my vision was blurring badly. I knew something was very wrong, so I went to a doctor. The news was not good, for my blood sugar was 596 mg/dl (normal is less than 99 mg/dl), and my blood pressure was rising out of control. The doctor gave me medication for diabetes and told me to lose weight and to exercise. I had appointments with him every two weeks and my weight went up and down like a roller coaster. I found any physical exercise difficult. His recommendations were to eat more fruit and vegetables. I felt lost, with little direction.

Finally, I asked for a referral to a nutritionist after several months of seeming to sink in a sea of hopelessness. My doctor refused to give me one! He again told me to just eat less and exercise more. Yeah, right, I thought. I'd tried to do that and failed so many times I lost count. I became convinced that somehow a nutritionist was my only shot at winning the war I was steadily losing. I demanded that he give me a referral. He acquiesced and gave me a referral to Judy. Days before my first appointment with this unknown lady, I felt a great deal of apprehension. I knew I was going to have to make a major lifestyle change and, that was very scary! Yet, an odd little bubble of optimism gamely bobbed around amid my anxiety and apprehension.

Prior to my appointment, I made a list of what I hoped to accomplish.

1. I wanted control of my life.

2. I wanted to like myself.

3. I wanted to feel good again, to be healthy.

4. I wanted to control my blood sugar and blood pressure without constant medication. I had watched a friend collapse and die of related problems while relatively young.

5. I wanted to stop running from relationships.

I had a gut feeling (no pun intended) that Judy and I would be able to do something with my life, my fears, and my failures. I realized that I was going to have to make the changes, but Judy would be my support and my coach while I learned to do it myself. Those first two weeks were a scary time. I found exercise machines boring and frustrating. Judy just kept encouraging me to find some form of exercise, suggesting walking and swimming. With her support I kept working at it.

I was making a *lot* of changes. The biggest change of all was that I started avoiding all milk and cheese (I hadn't expected this at all). I am now convinced that my success is directly linked to this key element. During my first follow-up visit, after two weeks, I was ecstatic to learn that I had lost seventeen pounds. I could do it! I felt a big chunk of power and control coming back to my life.

But this fleeting glimpse of victory was hard to hang onto. I had so much to lose; I found it a little depressing if I looked at the big picture. I saw my changes as accommodating a "diet," rather than making lifestyle changes. Judy kept encouraging me.

I was surprised to find that I really enjoyed walking as a form of exercise. It took time to build up my endurance, and to finally walk one mile was a major accomplish-ment. I continually challenged myself to increase my time and the distance, and I found that even after pushing myself to up my limits, I was a little less sweaty and a little less sore as time went by. Exercise was a tremendous help in making my lifestyle change. I just had to find what I enjoyed doing and then go and do it!

If I had been told two years ago that I would now weigh 180 pounds less, be able to effortlessly walk six miles a day and enjoy it, be healthy and strong, be married to a wonderful woman, and finally like myself for who I am, I would have laughed outright. Sure, let's just sell some more snake oil to the gullible! However, all these things have come true. I did it by myself; I won the war with myself. I accomplished all this with Judy's knowledge and guidance, and her caring and compassion.

Thanks, Judy, for everything. Thanks for my life!

Chapter 2

How Do I Begin?

Have you reached a point where you are convinced that it is impossible for you to lose weight? Or have you lost weight, only to have it creep right back on? Have you given up trying, believing that you're probably always going to be defeated and doomed to overeating? Have you finally decided that you must do something, *anything*, to get control of your overeating? Of your life?

Did you know that not every "weight-challenged" person is automatically an over eater?

What if there were some effective *and* attainable answers to your weight issues, answers no one has ever told you about? Are you really ready to take control of your life if you just could? Are you *truly* interested in losing weight— the sensible way? If you are, then read on, because The New E.A.T. and Be Healthy contains the necessary steps for you to not only finally *lose* that weight, but to *keep* it off.

Still reading? Good! You are about to discover a new approach that is different than any "commercial weight-loss program" you've ever heard about. This approach will help you learn how to determine your current eating patterns and evaluate them. It will help you learn how to tailor your eating patterns (not some *one-size-fits-all-doesn't-matter-if-you-hate-cottage-cheese* set of eating patterns) to fit basic nutritional principles. You will be able to eat "real" food with your family both at home and while dining out. You will learn how to successfully balance your eating, your attitude and your training (exercise). And, most importantly, you will learn the difference between *weight* loss and *fat* loss.

I will enter into a success-oriented partnership with you, fulfilling my part by becoming your "eating coach" and trainer.

You must take responsibility for your half of this contract, but I will guide you through the process of accomplishing that goal.

You must first determine whether or not you are willing to finally take control of your life. Losing weight is an active, ongoing process—a positive change in your approach to relating to food. This process of lifestyle change is what The New E.A.T. and Be Healthy is all about.

Many overeaters are "experts" on losing weight; their downfall comes in the battle of not gaining back the weight. Keeping weight off is the most difficult part of any weight loss program, the area of accomplishment that eludes so many people. Here is where the successful "loser" makes a paradigm shift in their thinking about losing weight. Most people who have a problem controlling their food intake consider losing weight an all-or-nothing proposition. They are either *on* a diet or they are *off* a diet. They have either been *good* or *bad* with regard to food in any given day. One or the other—with no middle ground in between. These people are counting--calories, grams, exchanges, or another measure--with a vengeance. Or they are eating everything that doesn't move,—compulsively, until it is gone.

There is a comfortable, satisfying middle-of-the-road area that they have never known, or have forgotten long ago. Together we will find that successful area of your life. Are you willing to restructure your ideas about eating? Are you willing to give up the belief that you will always be going on or falling off a diet? Are you willing to restructure your beliefs about your weight?

If you've believed that your weight is the root cause of all your problems, then you've probably also believed that your failure to remain on a successful diet has been keeping you from having all the "good" things you want in life. Have you ever said to yourself, "If I can just lose weight, then I will -- (fill in the blank!)" What would you fill in the blank with? Be happier? Get promoted? Get married? Be more popular?

The truth is this: your weight problem is generally just a reflection of what you eat and how many calories you burn (or fail to burn) over time. To realistically take control of your life, you need to recognize and accept that a resolved weight problem will not be a magic launching pad to catapult you into that "perfect life" that may have seemed to elude you for so long. Weight lost or gained has no magical value by itself to make your fantasies come true or self-destruct. But learning how to take control of your life, cutting the power that food, or any other external influence, holds over you, can help you move on to realizing your dreams.

Learning to keep weight off is an *attainable*, ongoing life-style process. I know this firsthand because I have a weight problem. My weight will always be a potential problem area for me, but it is an area I have learned to control and manage. Let me share my story with you.

"They" say pictures are worth a thousand words. What do my "before" and "after" pictures tell you about my weight?

BEFORE

AFTER

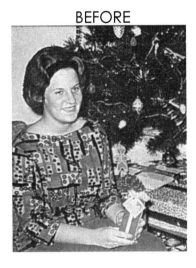
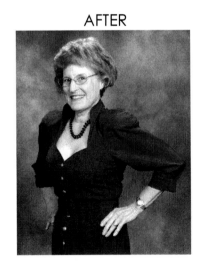

I was a normal weight at birth and on throughout my childhood, but I started putting on weight in adolescence. I had always been a tomboy, but when I became interested in boys and making myself look attractive, I also became a lot less active. Although I was still consuming the same amount of food that I had learned to eat, my reduced activity level could no longer burn up the excess calories, and my weight started going up. I was raised in a household with balanced meals and good, healthy snacks, yet (thanks to my father) we always had desserts. After school I would come home feeling like I was starving. My mother always offered fruits and vegetables, but they were never appealing to me. I just had to wait her out, for it was only a matter of time until I could have what I wanted.

That "time" would come just as soon as my mother left the house between five and six p.m. to meet my father's commuter train. As soon as she drove off, I would raid the cookie jar. Next, I would devour anything else I could find that might help stave off my seemingly unbearable hunger. Later, I would sit down to dinner with my family as if nothing had ever happened. I was certain that my misdeeds were never noticed, but I think now that my mother always knew. As a mother myself, I can tell if one of my youngsters has been into something. I believe it is that sixth sense that comes with being a mother!

During my last two years of high school, I gained fifteen extra pounds. Our family doctor cut right to the chase as he said, "You know, Judy, you really ought to lose some weight," but I totally rejected his words. What did *he* know? I was attractive, I had a boyfriend and I was active in school. I was only unhappy when it was time to buy clothes, and I struggled to ignore that it was getting harder and harder to find something that looked really good on me. But how often do you have to go out and buy new clothes, right?

As I ended my high school years, I was just anxious to graduate and go off to college—be free to do what I wanted. I was more than ready to be grown up! I was so excited and self-confident about the prospects of getting out "on my own," that I just knew I would become the popular, successful, have-it-all college student I fantasized being. I entered the University of California in the fall of 1963, and my fantasies and expectations quickly came crashing down around me.

I did anything but study, telling myself that the ultimate *college experience* was really all about having a good time and freedom from parents. I was sure that good grades would somehow come, just like they always had. But everyone in the freshman class at U.C. was from the top of their senior classes, so good grades were much harder to earn than in my high school years. And that was only the beginning of my problems! Besides the academic pressure, I found it very difficult to live with a roommate. I always had my own room and now I had to learn to share my space.

I was a "little" overweight, and I no longer had the social life I was used to having. I felt quite miserable and began to seek comfort and solace in popcorn, pizza, and other snacks in addition to three regular dorm meals every day. By Christmas break I had gained a whopping twenty-five additional pounds. Now, I was really unhappy—and obese, too.

My poor mother couldn't believe the change in me when I went home and I heard about it! When I went back to college after the break, I went straight to the student health center for help. The state-of-the-art weight "treatment" at that time was a prescription for diet pills. I took them, tried to cut down on my eating, and managed to lose about fifteen pounds during the next several months. A small battle won, while I seemed to be losing the rest of the war. By the end of my first year of college, I had been put on probation, dismissed from the dormitory for bad grades, and had become hooked on diet pills. On top of this, I was still fat and unhappy, even though I was physically active biking everywhere, on campus and off.

Not wanting to flunk out of college, I decided to look for a new major. After a little deliberation and talking to a girl in my dorm, I switched to dietetics. It was a fortuitous choice.

My early nutrition courses demanded that I plan a nutritious diet by hand (there were no computer software programs then). What I learned, I applied directly to my own life. Over the next year I finally began to lose weight sensibly. Since college and my dietetic internship, I have spent the past 44+ years in a most satisfying and reward-ing career, teaching my clients what I had to learn and must still practice every day of my life—balancing what I eat and what I expend.

Chapter 3

The Balancing Act

The E.A.T. Model

Learning the art of balancing your attitudes about food and exercise will be the first goal we will set together. There are three factors involved in your body's ability to process nutrients to your benefit, and the "secret" to the perfect weight for you is to know how to balance them. These three factors are (E) eating, (A) attitude, and (T) training or exercise. I have used these three factors to create the E.A.T. model, a dynamic, ever-changing, completely individual and personal model for your success. I have mastered it and you can, too. This is a goal that is definitely "doable".

In the illustrations that follow, visualize this: we have a ball, and on top of the ball we are putting a board. We are then trying to balance a triangular shaped block on top of this "moving" platform.

The block has three sections, represented by the letters E, A, and T. These letters represent three very basic human behaviors we all have: eating, attitude and training (or exercise).

First, let's look at what I call a "fat-gaining" model. In the drawing, the triangular-shaped block represents you when the "E" (eating) section is the largest. Eating would be a very high priority for you. You may always be thinking about eating. You may eat large amounts of everything, and yet you are never satisfied—stuffed and miserable, but not satisfied.

The "A" (attitude) section represents a scenario where you feel overwhelmed. You are negative in your outlook, and you don't believe you can succeed in this area or others. You may feel so poorly about your inability to achieve a satisfactory weight that you feel like your whole life is being impacted by negative and detrimental factors out of your control.

The "T" (training) section is the smallest, because you feel you have little or no time for purposeful exercise. The result of this combination of factors is that we can't stay balanced on the platform and fat gain results.

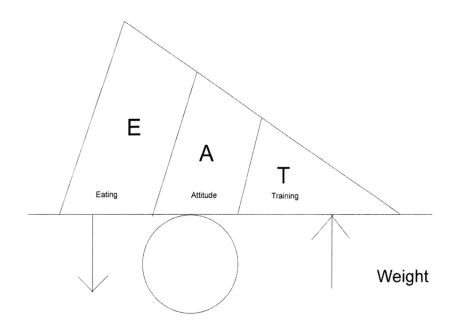

Fat Gaining Model

If this is a picture or model that fits your life, the most important question is this: how can you move from a fat-gaining to a fat-losing model?

In a "fat-losing model", our job in working together is to educate you on what you need to eat to be healthy, with food preoccupying your thought processes less than before. This includes virtually anything you like. These extras or "discretionary calories" are important to include in your eating pattern so you don't feel deprived.

For example, chocolate can be incorporated into your plan. In the past, you would probably feel it was not "okay" to have *any* chocolate. If you had one piece, you would have "blown" your entire "diet." Therefore, you might as well eat a whole pound! But when you are making optimal choices (lean protein, lots of vegetables and fruits, whole-grain breads and cereals), this "extra" chocolate can be part of the plan. Because you know it is "okay," you can be satisfied with a small amount. As you work in the E.A.T. model, you will learn to be aware of what you are eating and to enjoy eating foods you really like.

In the fat-losing model, the "A" (attitude) section is more positive because you will learn to balance all areas in your life. This is a win-win situation. You will not allow problems to tip you "off" balance. The demands or forces that we must learn to juggle will always be with us--for example, how to juggle work and family time, and how to relax and still make time for exercise.

The "T" (training) section is the most important in this "fat-losing model". It is regular and ongoing. You need to find an activity you enjoy so that you will continue it for the rest of your life. A wide variety of activities helps us deal with seasonal changes. For example, during the cold and wet winter, we still need to find something we will do on a regular basis. Training activities can be walking, biking, swimming or water exercises, or one—or more—of any number of active choices. Chapter 9 will give you more specific information on training and exercise.

Our objective, as a team, will be to help you learn how to balance these three components of your life at the same time. You may tend to fall back toward the board as you learn to adjust your E., A., and T. factors. You will learn how to find your equilibrium, or balancing point, regard-less of what life challenges you face.

For example, if you have a little extra to eat one day, you need to acknowledge that. Perhaps over the next several days you will be more attentive to portion sizes and limit extras. Because you are exercising regularly, you will not fall all the way over. In fact, increasing your exercise activity will be another way of burning off the extra calories. Learning the art of balancing these factors is the secret to maintaining weight loss.

You will learn what to eat for optimal nutrition and how many "extras," or discretionary calories, you will be able to add without upsetting your body's nutritional synergy. You will be aware of what you are eating, you will feel satisfied, and you will not feel deprived of the fun of eating the foods you find most pleasurable. Isn't it nice to know that you will not have to avoid or eliminate the foods you enjoy the most?

How do you move from a fat-gaining to a fat-losing model? This transition is the process you are just starting. First, you need to recognize where you are now. You do this by deciding how you would arrange the three components (your Eating, Attitude, and Training) to depict yourself as honestly as you can. The next step is to make some decisions, one step at a time, about the changes you need to make to bring the eating and training areas of your model into balance. You will learn more about this in the following chapters, but let's talk here about some of the other factors that impact your life.

In addition to your attitude (internal forces), there are also powerful external forces that affect your life as well. For example, you may be stressed at work, your children may be having trouble in school, or your parents may be ill and require help from you. The illustration below is our "transition" model".

The Transition Model

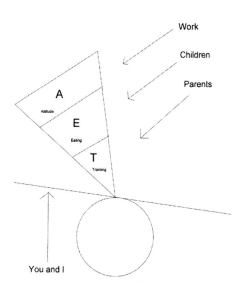

In this illustration, the attitude section is the largest, the result of a sense of being overpowered or overwhelmed. You and I will work as a team to push up on your block to strengthen your self-esteem and self-confidence. You may be managing to eat less and make better food choices, as well as getting more training or exercise by walking three times a week, but your weight-loss model is still not in balance. Your attitude is the out-of-balance factor to deal with now.

The three arrows directed toward the block represent three external forces pushing against you—such as your job, children, and parents. These external forces are having a major impact on your behavior. Since you can't simply wish these forces to go away, and you can't operate in a vacuum, you need to learn behavioral strategies that will help you achieve a counterbalance against them.

These behavioral strategies will help you realize that you are not overpowered; rather, you do have enough inner strength to take control of your life. If you are only able to control one new square foot of your life at a time, so be it. A square foot here and a square foot there is ground taken into your camp. This will empower you to have a more positive attitude.

There are many ways of problem solving for these forces so they will have less effect on what you are trying to do. For example, if you are overwhelmed with commuting to work, perhaps you can arrange to telecommute one day per week. If your children are fussy in the evening before dinner is ready, perhaps you can arrange for them to have a snack to hold them over to dinner; you may need a snack too, so you are not starving when you walk in the door. If your parents are still controlling your activities, you need to set some limits. As you accomplish these specific changes, you will be able to see things more clearly. This will help you evaluate your options to overcome the forces of the external obstacles.

After you have mastered one obstacle, another likely will replace it. But the victory of overcoming the first obstacle will help you see that you can overcome a second one too. This, indeed, is the challenge of living. You are going to learn how to meet each challenge creatively and positively, not just using food to cope with the problems that come your way.

I will show you, in the pages to come, how to balance all three of these areas at the same time. You will be aware of, and able to adjust, your thinking to positive attitudes about your weight and health goals, your ability to achieve them now and for the future. You will enjoy a more positive outlook when you are in control of your life. While I do suggest that you set your mind right now to adopt a take-no-prisoners-negotiate-no-compromise-attitude that nothing short of winning is what this objective will be all about, a little "teetering" back and forth on the board will not be cause for great alarm. The fine art of a steadfast balance is perfected through daily practice. Ask any Olympic gymnast.

The Maintenance Model

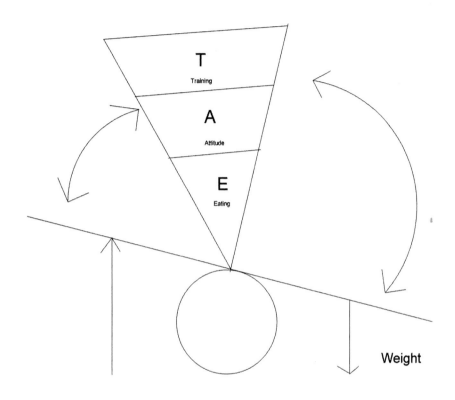

Chapter 4

Understanding the Difference between Weight Loss and *Fat* Loss

Please be prepared to make a paradigm shift here. Focusing on your scale's feedback can be quite counter-productive to achieving your desired body weight goal!

Losing excess body fat is more important than how much your scales say that you weigh. Really! Your scale can be your enemy, causing you to act irrationally, to get depressed, and to give up when the feedback is nega-tive. You must understand the difference between *weight loss* and *fat loss* to stay out of this self-defeating loop of thinking. At the beginning of any weight-loss program, most of us tend to be unrealistic about several things that we think will automatically happen once we are finally on the way to becoming leaner and trimmer. You would like to wave a magic wand and lose all of your excess weight yesterday, with little or no effort. Unfortunately, losing weight is sometimes a long process, requiring discipline at all times.

One of the first things you need to acknowledge and *really understand and believe* is that your scale is *not* your best friend in a weight loss effort. It often will lead you to believe that you are failing when, in fact, you are really winning. Whenever you step on a scale, you are measuring the total weight of all of your body's com-ponents. Your body (overall) is approximately 60% water, and shifts in your fluid "balance" can cause your scale weight to fluctuate rapidly. For example, if you were working outside on a hot day, you could "lose" one to three pounds— but you would have simply lost body water in perspiration. As soon as you respond to your natural thirst, those lost pounds would be added right back.

Your muscle mass by itself contains a lot of water—80% by weight. The body needs adequate quality protein (meat, fish, poultry, and dairy products) to supply the essential amino acids needed to build and repair muscle tissue. It needs this quality protein 24 hours a day, 365 days per year. You can actually lose weight faster the wrong way---by losing muscle, due to the loss of the associated water. You will tend to be more tired and have less energy as well. This is definitely not a smart idea! When you resume eating adequate protein, you can gain one pound for every 400 calories you eat to replace the lost muscle.

1 lb. muscle = 400 calories

One pound of body fat, on the other hand, contains 3,500 calories of stored energy. In order to lose one pound of excess body fat per week, you must (1) eat 500 calories fewer per day, or (2) exercise worth 500 calories per day, or (3) eat 250 calories per day less *and* exercise worth 250 calories per day. To double the weight loss to two pounds per week you must double all the above figures: (1) eat 1,000 calories fewer per day, or (2) exercise worth 1,000 calories per day, or (3) eat 500 calories fewer per day *and* exercise worth 500 calories per day.

One pound of fat consists of only 15% water by weight. Thus, the loss of fat is less influenced by shifts in fluid balance. You can feel thinner, with your clothes fitting looser, when you are losing excess body fat. Yet the changes on the scale are much slower. The water content of your body goes up with muscle. So you may actually weigh more or the same as you did initially. However, if you have made the changes: eating less, exercising more, or a combination of both, you will reduce your excess body fat.

Rather than using the scale as a means to rate your progress toward your desired goal, a more effective way to determine the loss of body fat is to take your body measurements each month. A loss in inches indicates a loss of body fat, as well as an increase in muscle toning. If your E.A.T. factors are in balance, much to your delight you will also note a decrease in your clothing size. If you were only weighing yourself on your scale, you might show nothing lost in pounds and become quite dis-couraged when you really had reason to be proud of yourself for becoming leaner and trimmer!

I recommend that you save one item of clothing that you wore at your heaviest. This will serve as a reminder of how far you have come and help reinforce your determination to never have to wear that item again. It is also a good idea to discard all intermediate-sized clothing items as you progress to your goal weight. You do not want to give yourself subconscious permission to regain the lost weight. Once you have arrived at your goal, you should have only the clothes you can wear at your ideal or best weight in your closet.

Use the following chart to note your measurements and goals.

Your Body Measurements

	Chest	Waist	Hips(7" below waist)
Date:	_____	_____	_____
Date:	_____	_____	_____
Date:	_____	_____	_____
Date:	_____	_____	_____

Determining Your Body Composition

One way of determining your body fat composition is with the use of skinfold calipers. This technique is quick, inexpensive, and non invasive. Your body frame size, as well as the percentage of muscle and percentage of fat you have in your body, can be calculated. These measurements can be repeated at intervals, and they will give you positive feedback on the behavioral changes you are making. It is important to use standardized techniques and age-corrected formulas in order to set a realistic body weight goal.

There are additional ways to measure body fat content. For a number of years the "gold standard" has been hydrostatic weighing. This method requires that you be weighed under water. When all factors are measured, this is the most accurate method, but it is not very practical for most people.

One of the most critical items, which should actually be measured, is your residual lung volume; this value should *not* be estimated. If you are interested in pursuing this technique, call your local university and ask for the adult fitness department. Costs can range from $50 and up, depending on the completeness of the assessment.

Another method which can be used is bioelectrical impedance. This technique measures total body water or fat-free mass; the percentage of fat is calculated by difference. Hydration levels, food intake, exercise, skin temperature, and menstrual cycle affect the accuracy of this method. Many types of scales utilizing this method are available for home use.

Chapter 5

Let's Look at What You Are Eating

We eat because our body needs energy, just as we put gas in our car when the fuel level is low. Depending on our bodies, the "octane" of our fuel can make a difference in how we burn our food, just as it does for the performance level of our cars. Our body has three main "areas" where energy or calories are stored. The largest storage area is fat with a capacity of around 140,000 calories. This is a normal level of fat storage, yet in overweight individuals this storage capacity increases dramatically. The second storage area, our lean body mass (protein), accounts for about 25,000 calories. Stored sugar/carbohydrate or glycogen in the liver accounts for a mere 1,200 calories.

These three terms—carbohydrate, protein, and fat—are what we call macro (large) nutrients. The fuel for our bodies is made up of a combination of these macro-nutrients. Our goal for your optimum program will be to combine these three macronutrients in an eating plan that best meets your individual calorie and nutrient needs.

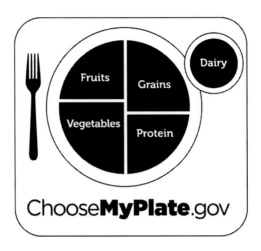

ChooseMyPlate.gov

The ChooseMyPlate diagram (choosemyplate.gov) of 2011 replaces the Food Pyramid from 1992 to help teach healthy eating. The goal of the graphic is to reinforce three principles:

1. **Variety:** Your mother was right. The more varied the food choices we make, the more likely we are to get all the nutrients we need.

2. **Moderation:** We should be able to eat anything we want as long as we do it in reasonable amounts. For example, if we have an overwhelming urge for chocolate, we should go ahead and have some. One ounce of chocolate counts as one serving of carbohydrate (CHO). If we consume the choco- late and take time to appreciate all of its sensory properties (odor, texture, etc.), we can satisfy the "urge" to OD (over-do) on chocolate. Because of all we've been told about good food/bad food and being overweight, we may believe we're "bad" if we have any chocolate at all. When we deprive

ourselves like this, we frequently end up eating an excessive amount.

3. **Proportionality:** This principle is important for balancing our food group servings in relation to each other. For example, some "experts" have taught that since meats and other protein sources have fat in them, they should be eliminated completely. This deprivation creates a tendency to eat more carbohydrates. Generally speaking, if your protein intake is not adequate, you will find yourself craving carbohydrate foods.

It is my observation that most people choose to embrace one concept at a time. For some time we were told to just avoid fat. Next, we were told to just eat carbo-hydrates. Obviously, neither one of these exclusive concepts has worked. Even though there is a tremend-ous drive to find a simple, easy solution for losing weight and maintaining that loss, the necessary principles for success are similar to what they have been for forty-plus years—we need to learn how to eat a balanced diet of a variety of foods. Let's learn more about how to do just that.

Macronutrients

Carbohydrate

Carbohydrate means "sugar" or "starch." Biochemically, a simple sugar is made up of two sugars hooked together. It is very easy for our bodies to break these two sugars apart and use them for energy. This is why you note the quick surge of energy after eating or drinking sugar. A starch, on the other hand, is made up of many sugars all hooked together. The amount of energy or calories derived from carbohydrates is 4 calories per gram. For example, a small apple contains 15 g (grams) of carbohydrates, or 60 calories (15 g x 4 = 60 calories).

Again, due to the teaching of many medical "experts," you may think you should greatly increase "complex carbohydrates" in your diet. Complex carbohydrates are vegetables, whole grain breads and cereals, and legumes (dry beans and peas). You do need to increase these complex carbohydrates, but not disproportionately to other food groups. Balance, as stated earlier, is the key to success for the E.A.T. program. For some individuals, a greater increase in vegetables with, perhaps, a decrease in bread, cereals, and legumes may be desirable.

Think about the foods you now eat that are your primary source of carbohydrates. List them below:

(1)   (6)

(2)   (7)

(3)   (8)

(4)   (9)

(5)   (10)

Have you listed fruit, fruit juice, vegetables, bread, cereal, muffins, potato, corn, rice, pasta, cooked dry beans, and milk? Both cooked dry beans and milk also supply a good amount of protein, but milk also supplies fat unless it is skim/nonfat or 1 % fat. Also included are items like cookies, cake, pie, ice cream, yogurt, and soft drinks.

Insulin is a hormone or chemical produced by your body which helps you derive energy from the carbohydrate foods you eat. Your pancreas produces this important hormone/chemical, releasing the right amount of insulin for the amount of available sugar, or carbohydrate, that you are eating. Visualize that insulin needs to match up with sugar to get inside the cell where energy is made. This combination is much like a key that we would use to open a door. Likewise, the cell is like the door. Each cell has receptor sites, which are like the lock. Our goal in helping you design your best eating pattern is to determine the amount of sugar or carbohydrate, that will allow you to feel good while unlocking your fat cells. This stored fat will then be used for energy. Let's go on to our second category.

Protein

Protein is made up of amino acids, which are the building blocks of muscle tissue. Bio-chemically, a protein looks a lot like a "slinky toy"—cylindrical in structure with amino acids coming off at different angles. Because of this more complicated structure, it takes our bodies longer to break down and use a protein food for energy. High quality proteins are those that contain all the essential amino acids our bodies need. Our bodies cannot manufacture nine of these amino acids, so the quality and quantity of protein in our diet is very important.

The amount of energy or calories derived from protein is 4 calories per gram. For example, a nonfat protein source such as 1 oz. white tuna packed in water contains 6 g of protein, or 24 calories (6 g x 4 cal/g = 24 calories). Other sources of quality protein may contain large amounts of fat, which increases the calories markedly. One ounce of pork sausage with 11 g fat has the same amount of protein as the tuna, but contains a whopping 123 calories (6 g protein x 4 cal/g = 24 calories plus 11 g fat x 9 cal/g = 99)! More about fat later.

Think about the foods you eat that supply primarily high-quality protein. List them below:

(1)   (3)

(2)   (4)

(5)   (6)

Have you included beef, pork, lamb, chicken, turkey, fish, shellfish, eggs, peanuts, dry beans, peas, and milk?

Fat

Fat is important in our diet too. It is true that as a rule we eat too much fat—about 37% of our total calories. Many people should decrease the fat they are eating, but not severely or entirely. We do need some fat in our diet to supply us with fat-soluble vitamins (A, D, E) and essential fatty acids. And generally we feel more satisfied after having some fat, which also contributes considerable flavor to our foods.

The amount of energy or calories derived from fat is 9 calories per gram. This is more than twice as many as are contained in carbohydrates and protein! For example, a teaspoon of butter, margarine, or oil provides 5 g fat or 45 calories (5 g x 9 cal/g = 45 calories).

Think about the foods you eat most often that supply you with mainly fat calories. List them below.

(1)   (4)

(2)   (5)

(3)   (6)

Have you included butter, margarine, oil, salad dressing, mayonnaise, sour cream, avocado, bacon, nuts? If you have, then you are aware of obvious sources of fat in foods.

Many other foods, though, contain large amounts of hidden fat, including potato chips, fried foods, donuts, muffins, cream-based soup, ice cream, cookies, pie, pastry, desserts, etc. Most of us don't think about these hidden calories from fat. Our goal will be to decrease the calories you eat from fat—lowering the percentage of your overall intake of fat to 25% to 30% of your diet. This is a realistic and desirable goal for most people.

Some people are very concerned about fat and cholesterol, so they omit or severely limit the fat-containing, high-quality protein foods. This is a mistake, as we discussed earlier. For example, choosing lower-fat protein can save significant calories without compromising protein quality. Choosing 6-oz. of white tuna in water or shrimp (150 calories and 0 fat) instead of 6-oz. pork sausage (780 calories and 66 g fat) saves 630 calories.

Alcohol

A fourth category in our diet is alcohol. Alcohol is not a macronutrient since it supplies no necessary nutrients. Still, it has almost as many calories as fat (7 calories per gram). For example, 1 oz. of 100-proof distilled spirits (whiskey, gin, etc.) has 100 calories. List below the items you know that are a source of alcohol:

(1)   (3)

(2)   (4)

Have you included beer, wine, champagne, and cocktails? You will be learning more in the next chapter about how to choose foods to obtain all the nutrients you need daily. Remember that our goal is to determine the best combination of macronutrients to meet your body's needs.

Balanced Diet

Most foods or meals contain combinations of the three macronutrients (carbohydrates, protein, and fat). To make it easier for people to eat healthy, foods have been grouped according to similarities in their composition. Our goals should include minimizing sugars, fats, and alcohol. One fourth of our plate should include quality protein such as lean meat, fish, and poultry; this area may also include dry beans and peas, nuts and seeds. The dairy section includes foods that supply calcium and protein. Fruits and vegetables should comprise one half our plate. The remaining one fourth of our plate includes breads, grains, and cereal products. Following are examples of how combinations of macronutrients (carbohydrate, protein, and fat) can be used for a meal.

Balanced Food Combinations

Carbohydrate	+	Protein	+	Fat	=	Comb. Food
2 slices bread		2 oz. beef		2 tsp. marg.	=	sandwich
1 lg. flour tortilla		1 cup refried beans		fat is in beans	=	burrito
2 cups salad greens		2 oz. chicken breast		1 tbsp. dressing	=	entree salad

Chapter 6
The Unique You

You are a unique individual, and just like the rest of us, you probably find yourself most pleased with and trusting of those unique "things" that are designed just for you—not the one size/pattern/model that fits everyone else in the world. I have written this book to guide you into an individualized meal pattern that should best satisfy your needs.

In order to have a starting point or baseline for your personal model of successful eating patterns, we need to determine and record what you have been doing and are doing now. For that purpose, I have provided a Daily Food Journal for you to write down everything you eat for the next three days. Do not try to eat just what you think is "right." I want you to completely resist changing your habits and portions of food that you eat just because you are writing it down.

You will need to estimate portion sizes (tablespoons, cups, ounces, inches, etc.) as closely as you are able, not just listing "one serving" of this and that. One person's single serving of a particular food can vary greatly from another person's concept of a single serving of that same food.

You may feel that four scoops is a "single serving bowl" of ice cream (approximately 600 calories), while another person may feel one scoop (1/2 cup) is a serving, at about 150 calories.

Make sure you have a set of measuring cups from your kitchen, the 1/2 cup and 1 cup measure being the most helpful. Also make sure you have a set of measuring spoons, with the tablespoon being the most helpful. Now you're ready to begin writing down everything that you eat, estimating your portions based on these measures. You will want to actually measure your food portions for the first day. Meat, fish, and poultry portions are usually given in weight measure after cooking, for example, three ounces of cooked beef. A deck of playing cards (3.5" x 2-1/2" x 1/2") resembles this portion of *cooked* meat. So, for example, if your steak were four times the size of a playing card deck, you would indicate twelve ounces.

Don't leave anything out, no matter how much you might be tempted. The list will never be used as evidence in "diet" court to show hidden secrets about your unsuccessful eating habits. Rather, this list will be the starting point of how we design your personalized eating pattern.

When you eat a combination food, it is much easier to evaluate for macronutrients if you list the components separately. For example, instead of writing down "1 hamburger," you should list "1 large hamburger bun, 3 oz. meat patty, 1 tablespoon mayonnaise, 1 slice each onion, tomato, and leaf lettuce." Likewise, if you had a beef noodle casserole, try your best to estimate the contribution of the component parts. For example, if your recipe calls for six servings, you can divide all the ingredients by six to estimate your portion.

DAILY FOOD JOURNAL

FOOD EATEN   **AMOUNT**

Day 1:

DAILY FOOD JOURNAL

FOOD EATEN   **AMOUNT**

Day 2:

DAILY FOOD JOURNAL

FOOD EATEN   **AMOUNT**

Day 3:

FOOD GUIDE

Foods have been divided into groups based on similarities in macronutrients provided. Remember, the macronutrients are carbohydrate, protein, and fat. I have called this a Food Guide since it will show you how to make choices of the foods you like. It is important that the macronutrient composition stay about the same from one day to the next. Refer to the index for the complete guide.

Protein-Rich Foods (PRO)

The foods on this list supply an average of 6-7 grams of protein and varying amounts of fat; the average calorie content is 70 per ounce. You may use the chart in the Appendix to choose protein sources that are the lowest in fat. For example, if you want to have sausage for breakfast—which is high in fat at 11 grams per ounce of cooked sausage—you then can choose lower fat sources of protein throughout the rest of the day. For example, having two ounces of white water packed tuna and 1/2 cup low-fat cottage cheese will give you a total of 12.5 grams of fat, or an average of 2.5 grams fat per the five ounces total protein for the day. Another benefit of the above foods is that they are generally good sources of vitamins B-6, iron, and zinc.

Starch (CHO)

This group of foods includes breads, cereals, grains, and starchy vegetables. Each serving supplies about 70 calories with 15 grams of carbohydrate and 3 grams of protein. These foods supply starch (carbohydrate), protein, vitamins, and minerals. Whole grain products are good sources of fiber; they also contain thiamin, niacin, folate, vitamin E, iron, phosphorus, magnesium, zinc, and other trace minerals. Some products may be "enriched" (thiamin, riboflavin, niacin, and iron are added back after processing), but they tend to be lower in fiber. Other products, such as ready to eat cereal, may be fortified with additional nutrients. The fiber content in a food may be subtracted from the total carbohydrate *only* when the insoluble fiber is 5 g or higher to yield the net available carbohydrate. For example, a bran flake cereal label reads 22 g carbohydrate and 6 g fiber for 1 oz. or 2/3 cup. The available carbohydrate is 16 g or 1 CHO (22 g minus 6 g = 16 g).

Fruit (CHO)

This group of food supplies fiber when the whole fruit is consumed, rather than juice. One serving per day should be a good source of vitamin C; fruits high in this vitamin are marked with a (C) in the Appendix. One serving of fruit supplies 60 calories and 15 grams of carbohydrate. Since the carbohydrate content (15 g) is the same as for starch, you may be allowed to inter-change these servings. Some fruits are a good source of vitamin A; fruits high in this vitamin are marked with a (A) in the Appendix.

Vegetable (VEG)

The foods on this list are generally low in calories and you may eat them freely; one serving averages 25 calories with 5 grams of carbohydrate and 2 grams of protein. You should try to include a minimum of four servings daily, especially since they are generally important sources of fiber. Some vegetables are also good sources of vitamin C and vitamin A; they are noted with (C) and (A) respectively in the Appendix. When eaten fresh or when minimally cooked, the vitamin C and folate content will be preserved. Dark green vegetables are generally good sources of vitamin B-6, folate, and magnesium.

Milk Product (CHO + PRO)

The foods included on this list provide at least 250 mg. calcium per serving, in addition to magnesium and zinc. Milk products are good sources of protein, riboflavin, thiamin, and vitamins A, B-6, and B-12. Since both fluid and dry milk are fortified, they are also good sources of vitamin D. Milk products may serve as the primary source of protein and vitamin B-12 for people consuming a vegetarian diet. If you are not a milk drinker, your meal pattern will have to be adjusted for its macronutrient composition. For example, for each glass of milk you do not drink, you need to add 1 oz. of the protein-rich foods and one serving of starch or fruit. In addition, you need to choose alternate calcium sources (table follows), or you may need to take a calcium supplement. Each serving of milk product supplies about 80 calories with 12 grams of carbohydrate and 8 grams of protein.

Alternate Calcium Sources

The following foods supply 250 mg. calcium in the amounts indicated. The information on calories, carbohydrate (CHO in grams), protein (PRO in grams), and fat (FAT in grams) has been added to assist you in incorporating these foods into your meal plan.

TABLE: alternate sources of 250-mg. calcium

FOOD ITEM	CALORIES	CHO	PRO	FAT
2-1/2 oz. sardine with bones	105	0	12	6
1/2 c. canned salmon with bone	72	0	11	3
5 oz canned mackerel	160	0	24	7
9 oz tofu processed with calcium	207	5	22	13
4 oz almonds	668	23	23	59
¼ cup tahini (sesame butter)	356	13	10	32
2 c. baked beans	536	101	2	8
7 corn tortillas (masa harina)	469	90	15	8
5 medium oranges	295	72	7	2
1-1/2 c. cooked broccoli	69	13	7	0.6
1-1/2 c. cooked turnip greens	45	9	2	0.6
2 c. bok choy	40	6	5	5
2 c. cooked collard/dandelion greens	68	13	4	1.2
3 c. cooked kale/mustard greens	126	22	7	2
2 T. blackstrap molasses	86	22	0	0

FAT

The foods in this list provide a concentrated source of calories. Remember that fat supplies 9 calories per gram. Each serving supplies 50 calories and 5 grams of fat. Fats supply fat soluble vitamins A, D, and E, as well as linoleic acid, an essential fatty acid. Linoleic acid is called an essential fatty acid because it cannot be made in our body; we must obtain it in our food.

Fatty acids are the basic chemical units in fat. They are saturated, monounsaturated, or polyunsaturated depending on the amount of hydrogen they contain. A saturated fat is like a bus with all the seats filled; there will not be a lot of activity on that bus. A mono-unsaturated fat is like a bus with one seat empty; there will not be a lot of activity—only one person can get on or off. Polyunsaturated fat is like a bus with many empty seats; there will be a lot of activity on this bus. Saturated fat is considered the most harmful to the body. It is preferable to use both mono- and poly- unsaturated fats as much as you can. All dietary fats contain various amounts of these three types of fatty acids. Fats high in unsaturated fatty acids are good sources of vitamin E and linoleic acid. When mono or polyunsaturated fat is partially hydrogenated (made harder), its content of trans fatty acids is increased. Since we cannot metabolize or use these, you should choose a soft tub or liquid margarine where liquid oil is the first ingredient. Our goal for your meal plan will be to include a daily minimum of three servings added fats which are high in both polyunsaturated and monounsaturated fatty acids. Another goal will be to limit your caloric intake of fat content in all foods to 30% or less of your total daily calories. Instead of counting fat grams, make the most of your protein-rich food choices from those with the least amount of fat; some of your total protein choices may have medium amounts of fat. Thus, when minimal fat is used, you will automatically average 30% or less of total calories from fat without counting fat grams.

Sugars and Discretionary Calories (CHO)

Sugars supply mainly energy with few additional nutrients found in them. Many sweet treats that are so tempting also supply large amounts of fat. Since nearly everyone who wants to lose weight does not want to feel deprived, we will include some discretionary calories in your meal plan daily. These are divided into 150-calorie choices. Some examples include the following, while additional choices may be added in consultation with your personal Registered Dietitian.

Examples of Discretionary Calories (CHO)

1 oz. chocolate	½ oz. hard candy
2 oz. cake (2-in. square of 13 x 9)	1 oz. donut
1 oz cookie (depends on size)	1 oz. granola bar

2 oz. pie (1/16th of 9-in.)   4 oz wine

6 oz. average mixed drink   6 oz. wine cooler

12 oz. light beer

Use as Desired

A free food is one containing less than 20 calories or less than 5 g carbohydrate per serving. The following foods are examples of free foods and can be consumed as desired: sugar free gelatin, clear broth or bouillon, black coffee, tea, mineral water, club soda, sugar free carbonated beverages, pure spices and herbs, and sugar free popsicles.

Summary of Macronutrients per Food Group, per serving

(carbohydrate, protein, and fat are in gram amounts)

Food Group	calories	carbohydrate	protein	fat
Protein-rich (PRO)	70		7	4
Starch (CHO)	80	15	3	
Fruit (CHO)	60	15		
Vegetable (VEG)	25	5	2	
Milk Product (CHO+PRO)	80	12	8	
Fat and Oil	50			5
Discretionary	150	15	3	8

Choose My Plate Recommendations

PROTEIN-RICH (PRO)

4-6 oz. per day

1 oz. = 1 oz. cooked *lean* beef, pork, chicken, or turkey

= 1 oz. prepared meat with 4 grams fat or less per oz. and 6--7 grams of protein

= 1 egg (limit yolks to four per week if cholesterol elevated)

= 1/3 of a 12.3 oz. box reduced fat tofu

= 1/2 cup cooked dry beans or legumes

= 2 Tbsp. nut butter

= 1/3 cup nuts

= 1/4 cup seeds

STARCH (CHO)

> **6 or more servings/day; whole grain choices are high in fiber**

1 serving   = 1 slice bread (1 oz. in weight)

= 1 small tortilla (fajita size)

= 1/2 cooked cereal, rice, pasta, corn, potato, cooked dry beans and peas

= 1 oz. dry cereal (check label for portion size)

= 2/3 oz. crackers or pretzels

= 1/2 small bagel, English muffin or hamburger bun

= 3 cups popped popcorn (no fat)

FRUIT (CHO)

> **2 or more servings/day; fruit is high in fiber and may supply vitamin A or C**

1 serving   = 6 oz. juice

              = 1/2 cup fruit

              = 1/4 cup dried fruit

Good Vitamin A sources: apricots, cantaloupe, and papaya

Good Vitamin C sources: orange, grapefruit, cantaloupe, kiwi, lemon, papaya, strawberry, tangerine

VEGETABLE (VEG)

> **4 or more servings per day; source of vitamins A and C**

1 serving   = 6 oz. juice

              = 1/2 cup vegetable, cooked or raw

              = 1 cup raw leafy vegetables (salad greens)

Good vitamin A sources: beet or other greens, carrot, kale, parsley, peppers, pumpkin, green onion, spinach, winter squash, sweet potato or yam, tomato

Good vitamin C sources: broccoli, Brussels sprouts, cabbage, cauliflower, peppers, snow peas

MILK PRODUCTS (CHO + PRO)

2 to 3 servings/day; source of calcium and quality protein

1 serving = 1 cup 1% or nonfat milk

= 1 cup fortified soymilk (10-13 g carbohydrate 8-10 g protein)

= 1 cup reduced fat goat milk

= 1 cup nonfat plain yogurt

= 1-1/2 oz. low fat cheese (4 g fat or less/oz.)

FATS AND OILS

3 to 6 tsp. a day

One teaspoon of fat contains 5 grams of fat. The above allotment includes any added fat used in preparation or at the table. For processed foods and high fat meats (sausage, hot dogs, etc.) subtract 1 teaspoon added fat for each 5 grams fat over the average fat content per ounce cooked weight lean protein (4 grams). For example, since 1 oz. cooked pork sausage contains 10 grams fat, you would subtract 1 tsp. of your added fat for the day (10 g fat in sausage − 4 g fat in 1 oz. *lean* protein = 6 g fat or 1 tsp.)

1 tsp. fat = 1 tsp. butter, margarine, oil, mayonnaise

= 2 tsp. salad dressing

= 2 Tbsp. sour cream

= 1 Tbsp. cream cheese

Current Eating Habits

Now it is time to evaluate your usual eating habits. Review your three days' records and count up the number of servings of the various food groups. Remember to look for hidden fats and sugars. Summarize your results as in the example below.

Food	Amount	Food Group
Cake donut	2	2 discretionary (high fat)
Coffee, cream/sugar	2 Tbsp/2 tsp.	1 fat; ½ discretionary
Cheeseburger	1 small	2 starch and 1—1/2 oz. meat (high fat)
French fries	Small	1 starch/3 fat
Soda	Large	2 discretionary
Frozen dinner	<300 cal.	1—1/2 oz. meat, 1 starch, 1 vegetable
Wine	4 oz.	1 discretionary
Popcorn, microwave	1 bag	4 starch
Soda	12 oz.	2 discretionary

Let's work through an example here for comparison to a target eating pattern:

In summary then	Your goal was:	You consumed:
Meat/alternate	4-6 oz.	3 oz.
Milk	2-3	0
Starches	6+	8.5
Vegetables	4	1
Discretionary	1	7.5
Fats	3	4+

In our example, it is easy to see that you did not eat the recommended ounces of protein or quantity of vegetables. You ate no fruit and had a lot of extra discretionary calories (7.5 servings x 150 cal/serving = 1,125). You also had no choices from the milk group.

Our goal will be for you to learn new eating patterns that you can live with long-term. To successfully do so, we will want to design a combination of food servings that will effectively silence all of the food cravings you have been besieged with in the past. Your eating plan must include an adequate amount of high quality protein, at least 4-6 oz. per day, and 2-3 servings of dairy products. You will also need a minimum of four servings of vegetables each day. To keep your fat intake low, you will work toward limiting added fat to four servings or less. It is obvious that you will also cut out extra fat and sugar by limiting your discretionary calories.

If you will not or cannot drink milk, you will need to make some additional adjustments in your meal plan. You will need to include some calcium-rich foods, and I usually recommend adding a calcium supplement as well. I generally suggest a product containing calcium and magnesium with Vitamin D3. The total amounts of these minerals in three tablets should be approximately: 1,200 mg. calcium, 400 mg. magnesium, and 400 IU Vitamin D3. Females need these amounts daily, while males need two-thirds the above amounts, or two tablets per day. You can also look for other sources of calcium, such as fortified juices, chewable forms of calcium, etc.

Since milk supplies 12 grams of carbohydrate and 8 grams of protein per cup, you must also make adjustments in the macro nutrient composition of your meal plan. You would count 1 cup milk as 1 starch or fruit (CHO) and 1oz. protein-rich (PRO) serving. Refer to the macro nutrient chart earlier in this chapter to assist you in making these adjustments.

A revised meal pattern may look like this:

Food	Amount	Food group
Cake donut	1	1 discretionary
Lean ham	1 oz.	1 oz. meat
Coffee, black	1 cup	0
Nonfat milk	1 cup	1 milk
Sugar substitute	1 packet	0
¼ lb. hamburger	1	3 oz. meat and 2 starch
Side salad	2 cups	2 vegetable
Low calorie dressing	½ packet	1 fat
Diet soft drink	12 oz	0
Frozen dinner	<300 calories	1—1/2 oz meat and 1 starch, 1 vegetable
Sliced tomato	1	1 vegetable
Mineral water with juice	12 oz./ 1/2 cup fruit juice	1 fruit
Light popcorn	¼ bag	1 starch
Low fat cheese	2 oz.	1 milk

In summary, then, you consumed:

5.5 oz. meat/alternate

2 milk

4.5 starches

1 fruit

4 vegetables

1 fat

1 discretionary

Now add up the food group totals to see what you have included in macronutrient servings: 7.5 oz. protein [5.5 oz. + 2 oz. for milk] (PRO), 4 vegetables (VEG), 7.5 starch, including fruit and milk (CHO). Since these supply 12--15 g carbohydrates, they may be interchanged. The total also includes 1 each discretionary and fat. I have limited the added fat, since a donut was included at breakfast and a fast food hamburger at lunch. You saved 925 calories from the earlier menu by limiting your discretionary calories.

Since you increased the servings of high quality protein and vegetables, the increased fiber content should stave off any significant hunger pangs. Designing a meal pattern with the best combination of macronutrients for you can be quite challenging. You may need the assistance of a Registered Dietitian to help you get started. Do not hesitate to seek a referral to one, as you will benefit from their experienced advice. Success—once and for all—is your goal, so draw upon all of the qualified experience you are able to in order to create the healthiest, best tasting, livable eating plan you can.

In the meal plan designed above, the total calories per day average 1,200; the macro nutrient composition is about 110 g carbohydrate, 80 g protein, and 45 g fat. Should your calorie level fall below 1,200, you need to incorporate a good multiple vitamin/mineral supplement into your daily intake. The supplement should supply approximately 100% of the RDI (Recommended Dietary Intake).

I frequently suggest Centrum® or its generic equivalent. An additional caloric deficit (calories burned) will be created by regular aerobic exercise, which will be discussed in a later chapter.

Chapter 7

The Magic of The Mirror

When you look in the mirror or in storefront window reflections, how do you see yourself? Do you really see yourself as you are today? Or do you see your body of twenty years earlier? Or perhaps only your head and shoulders? Do you avoid looking at your reflection at all?

When we have a weight problem, our eyes and brains can play tricks on us. Somehow we reason that if we don't "see" the problem, perhaps it really doesn't exist. I would like you to enlist the help of a friend or family member with the following task. I want you to roll out on the floor lengths of butcher paper on which you are going to trace the outline of your body. When you do this exercise, it is helpful to wear minimal clothing. Center your body on top of the paper with your arms at your side and your legs extended. The helper is to trace an outline of your body. Be sure to date this drawing. I suggest that you repeat the tracing, on the same paper, every two months, using different color ink and dating each one. You should see your body getting smaller and smaller as you get leaner. This gives you concrete evidence that your image is changing.

Another exercise for working on your image is to look through photographs of yourself and find one that looks like you want to look. This should be placed where you can easily see it. You goal is to "see" yourself looking more like the image in the picture every day.

Pictures can help us see our bodies realistically. Again, enlist the help of a friend or family member. Take full body photographs of your body from first one side then the other, then front and back. These body shots are solely for your personal use. You will be able to use them when developing your specific reasons for losing weight (see Chapter 8). In addition, since you may not have a full-length mirror, you may not be used to looking at your whole body. I remember a woman who did not realize what she looked like from the backside until she saw her picture. She was horrified with what she saw and very motivated to change. She was only used to looking at herself from the neck up. For her, it was as though the body below belonged to someone else.

You need to understand your weight problem and how you see yourself. Outside influences do impact our perceptions. The home environment we grew up in also has a tremendous impact. You may have been in a household where only high fat, unhealthy food was served. Your parents may have had a weight problem, and your resources were limited to what they provided for you. Maybe you were in a stressful environment where food became your only source of comfort. You need to know that there are many contributing factors why we eat and consequently how we come up with what we think is a *realistic* weight goal, while, in fact, it may be an *unhealthy* weight goal. It is important that you understand that *it is not healthy to be <u>either</u> too thin or too heavy.*

Your Weight Problem

We live in a society where social and family situations sometimes define our perceptions for us. Unfortunately, your perceptions may be influenced by outside factors giving you unrealistic views.

Everywhere you look, there are messages promoting the "ideal" body-one that is actually too thin. Billboards, magazines, and the media promote a body that is many times achieved by unhealthy choices. Many of these "ideal" body types eat only 800 calories per day with an exercise regimen that includes 1 to 2 hours of vigorous exercise per day. I don't know about you, but <u>I am certain</u> there has to be a better way! Working together, we will create realistic goals that fit your individual lifestyle.

I hope you are reading this book because you want to modify your weight for *yourself.* Lifelong battles are lost when they are fought for someone else. If there is not a personal investment, long term goals and visions become clouded with discouragement and hopelessness. Sometimes friends and significant others put unnecessary pressures on us to do what *they* believe is best for us.

Have you ever been offered a reward for losing weight... trip...new clothes? Initially, you think this is the motivation you need to begin your diet, but sooner or later you are back to square one again. Someone, well-meaning of course, may say to you "Are you sure you want whipped cream on your mocha?" or they may say as much with the disdainful look they give you as you order a piece of pie instead of a vegetable smoothie! Many times, our response is one of rebellion instead of empathy: "I will have a double mocha, with *extra* cream please!" or "Don't look at me like that, I will order what I want to!" and thus, the battle continues.

As you take responsibility for your own life, your personal satisfaction will be a reward far more valuable than a weekend trip or new outfit. Let's get started on some practical guidelines. Imagine that there are actually three different components within you: you, the 'adult'; you, the 'parent'; and you, the 'child'. You have the choice, in your relationship with others, to decide which component will dominate. Unfortunately, one usually responds automatically without thinking through what type of response is most appropriate. In your weight loss efforts you need your *adult* in charge. This is the person who can reason and act rationally in a given circumstance. When a well-meaning person tells you what to do, they are 'parenting' you. It takes a great deal of maturity for you not to react as the *child*. This may sound elementary, yet it takes practice, practice, and then some more practice in order for you to change your automatic responses. But take heart; it can be done!

As the days and weeks of your weight loss journey pass, be conscious of your responses. If you sense a pattern of acting like a *child* you can work to modify your behavior. This is an important step in taking responsibility. Not only will this help you make intelligent choices for yourself, but also it can help you in your interpersonal skills in your work environment or social situations. Continue to ask yourself: "Am I acting as an adult, parent, or child?"

It is now time to make a realistic assessment of your body type. Remember that there are no miracle cures! If you are five feet tall, losing weight will not make you taller. You are laughing, but believe me; I have had many clients who have had totally unrealistic expectations! If you are a large person who has a "stocky" build, your muscle mass is generally higher than average, and you will tend to weigh more and yet look your best. Remember that muscle tissue is very compact, and it is also high in water content (80%). Thus, if you have more lean body mass (muscle), you will weigh more on the scale. Has anyone ever been surprised to learn what you weigh? Or, have you been told that you carry your weight very well? This may mean that you have a higher proportion of muscle tissue than other people do.

If you can pinch more than a 1-inch thickness of skin and fat at your waist, your body fat composition may be excessive. Your goal should always be to reduce your body fat composition to a realistic level for your age and sex. When that is achieved, looking and feeling good will be an automatic byproduct. Registered dietitians, personal trainers, and health clubs can assist you with measures of your frame, muscle, and body fat content. But always remember one important thing:

In our attempt to lose weight, many times we determine our success by the number we read on the scale. For years, this has been the way people gauged their success. It is time to make a paradigm shift. The number on the scale is not the important issue; it is the *body fat content*. When you are appropriately lean, your overall health improves. Many times excess body fat contributes to an increased incidence of sickness and disease. When your body is at the appropriate weight, your quality of life improves. The risks of chronic sickness and disease will greatly decrease as your blood sugar and blood fats normalize. For instance, people who have had problems with high blood pressure usually see decreased levels. The many benefits of a healthy lifestyle, including greater mental productivity, far outweigh the consequences of an unhealthy body.

Maintaining your weight becomes easier as you become leaner. It is a very complex process, but start to visualize your fat cells being emptied of fat to a lower level. Once they have attained this level, they are no longer under the constant pressure to immediately fill up again. Bear in mind, there are many dynamics involved in weight control, and there are no set answers for any one person. It truly is a juggling act that involves not only your eating habits, but your training and attitude as well. The good news is, once you have learned to keep all these components in balance, you can essentially eat anything you want, within reason.

Optimal health requires proper eating, attitude and training. Your *attitude* plays a significant part in this process. The next chapter will give you keys to unlock the door to a fresh attitude that will enable you to achieve your goals and maintain a healthy lifestyle.

Chapter 8

Why Do You *Really* Want to Lose Weight?

At this point in your reading, you are, I assume, beyond wanting a "magic pill" remedy. You recognize that you need sound information that will help you learn how to lose your excess weight and *keep* it off, especially while eating the foods you like.

Your motivation to change must come from within. Our task is to identify what specific long-term goals you would like to accomplish. We will be discussing how to identify those goals and then stay focused on them day to day.

I would like you to write down *very specifically* why you want to lose weight. After some serious thought, see if you can come up with twelve specific *true goals and desires* that are very personal to you. For example, do not write, "I want to look better." This is not specific enough. You may know what you mean by that, but if you are tired and faced with a plate full of donuts, you may not care what you look like at the moment. Some ideas that might stimulate your thinking follow: Explain how you think your life will be different if you lose weight; state how losing weight will help you accomplish other goals you have in life; explain how you think a loss of weight will change how other people treat you; state specifically how your health will improve.

If you are like most people, you will have trouble with this exercise. You will probably tend to write down a few general reasons and feel frustrated. It is not important why others think you should lose weight. Following are some examples to get you started:

1. I want to reduce my blood pressure.

2. I want to walk up two flights of stairs without becoming short of breath.

3. I want to wear my jeans comfortably and to be able to zip them while standing.

4. I want to wear my blouse/shirt tucked in.

5. I want to rollerblade with my children.

6. I want to lower my cholesterol.

As time goes along, feel free to modify your list. For example, one day a client said to me, "My slip fell off!" Literally, her slip had fallen off her hips and down around her ankles (fortunately at home). She had lost enough body fat that her clothes size changed before she realized it—a dramatic illustration of positive change. Some of her initial goals had been met and to have her slip fall off had not been one of them! It was time to revise and add some new reasons. As you accomplish one goal, you can add another. For example, when your jeans fit, replace that goal with "I want to wear shorts."

Now complete your specific reasons you want to reach your ideal size:

WHY I WANT TO REACH MY IDEAL SIZE

1.

2.

3.

4.

5.

6.

7.

8.

9.

10.

11.

12.

Now we will review how you can use these reasons to reinforce your motivation or drive to change. I suggest that you transfer these reasons to a small card, which you can easily carry with you at all times. Read it first thing in the morning when you get up. Then, re-read it before you put something in your mouth. Last, before you retire, read it one more time for the day.

This exercise is to help you stop and *think* before you start for the day and as you finish your day, and especially before you eat. You are delaying your decision to eat—time enough to make the best choice. You need to ask yourself, "Am I really hungry? Or do I want to eat right now because I'm frustrated, depressed, upset, angry, etc?" If the latter is the case, that is often followed by "I *deserve* to eat something to make myself feel better." Later we will talk more about these behavioral issues, but for now, reading these twelve reasons regularly can help you refocus and maintain your motivation.

Earlier I asked you to save one of your largest size items of clothing: a blouse and skirt, a dress, or a shirt and slacks. As you progress towards your thinner self, please give away, donate, or simply discard all of your intermediate size clothing. Keeping a closet full of various clothing sizes—*just in case*—gives your subconscious "permission" to regain weight at some future point in time. You must be firmly committed to losing your excess weight and fat once and for all. Burning bridges is not always a wise thing to do in life, but it is here! Get rid of all your former sized clothes, too (except the one largest example you're going to keep for future motivation).

Trying on your largest item of clothing periodically is positive reinforcement. Your motivation will be enhanced; you may wonder how you could have ever worn that size. The important thing now is that you must be determined to never wear it again. Once you have maintained your ideal weight for six months or longer, you will tend to forget your former size.

Your personal motivation *must* come from within you. My personal story, or stories of other successful patients, will not guarantee that you will do well. *You* must be determined to do well. *You* have to choose to want to change your eating habits. *You* have to choose to want to change your exercise habits. The information you're learning and the exercises you're doing in this book will help you make those choices. You can do it!

Every time you re-read your "12 Reasons" list, you will be constantly reinforcing exactly what *you* want to do. You will be concentrating on the *positive* reasons you are making lifestyle changes so that you can lose that unwanted weight.

When taken together, each of these specific goals are part of a much larger goal. For example, losing 2 pounds a week may not seem like much of an accomplishment if you are viewing it in the "short-term". However, think about the dramatic long-term changes-- 2 pounds a week translates to 104 pounds in a year! Now, *that is* a tremendous accomplishment!

You can achieve your "impossible dream" just by being successful a little bit at a time. Persistently working at changing small behaviors will build the bridge you need to reach your very "possible" dream. Then it will no longer be a dream, will it? It will be a reality.

Chapter 9

What About Exercise?

Exercise is the most critical lifestyle change you must make to achieve your desired lean body size. Surprisingly, exercise is even more important than what you eat.

Stop groaning, I'm going to help you see this as a truth that will work wonders for you!

As you think about choosing an exercise or activity to include in your E.A.T. model, I want you to think in terms of what you think you *would still enjoy doing a year from now*. You will be more apt to continue an activity that easily fits into your schedule and your interests. For many people, a variety of activities (called cross training) will help to prevent boredom. Cross training also works more muscle groups than a single form of activity.

Let me pretend to listen in on what I believe you're thinking right now. "Exercise? I'm busy all day. I'm constantly walking on my job. I bend, I lift, and I hustle all day long. I'm tired when I get home. Give me a break!" And I believe you probably do many, if not all and more, of these activities at your job or at your home. The only problem with *these activities* is that they do not last long enough to raise your heart rate and maintain it for a sufficient length of time. If you question this, take your heart rate when performing these tasks. If it increases adequately *and* you are able to maintain it at the elevated level for twenty minutes or more, you may be able to justify your daily work "activity" for your exercise.

Exercise is Critical

The secret to effective exercise is that it must be aerobic, or "using oxygen". In practical terms, the effectiveness of any form of exercise can be judged by simply measuring your heart rate while performing the activity. Your heart rate reflects the volume of oxygen you are taking into your body.

Remember that your body is an engine, and you have extra fat stored away that you want to be converted to energy. Aerobic exercise raises the "RPM" of your engine, or the rate at which you burn calories. When you reduce your daily intake of "new" calories, your body will hunt out and use its fat stores (old surplus calories) for the fuel demanded by your increase in aerobic activity.

Some of you who are over-fat may have very efficient engines. This is both good and bad news for those who have been struggling to reduce their body fat. Your engine burns fuel so efficiently, less fuel is required for your daily energy needs. Don't you wish your car's engine ran like that? However, much of what you eat is not required for energy output every day, and so it is stored for future reserves. In the event of disaster or famine, you have an advantage. You would be the one who could survive longer without food since your fat stores would supply the needed calories. You are also the one who says, "I can just look at food and gain weight."

Store vs. Use Fat?

It is incredibly easy for some people to *store* fat. Yet, when it comes time to *use* the stored fat, the fat cell does not want to open up and let the stored energy out. This is one reason exercise is so important. Exercise seems to affect the receptor sites on the surface of your body's cells. For each of us, there is a "best" combination of eating and exercise that will allow excess fat to be lost. Our job is to help you find that magic or "best" combination.

Let me first tell you how to take your pulse rate. Usually, the easiest site for you to use is your radial pulse. The radial artery runs along the inside of your wrist in a direct line from your thumb. Take the first and second fingers of one hand and put the tips of those fingers on top of the line running up your wrist from your thumb.

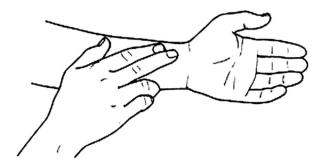

You will need to put a slight amount of pressure in your fingertips. When you feel a "pulsing" on a regular basis, you are feeling your pulse rate. Every time you feel a pulse, your heart valves are opening and closing. You will use your pulse rate to measure the effectiveness of your exercise.

First, place a watch or clock with a second hand in front of you to measure your pulse rate while you are in a state of resting. Second, place your fingers as on the area of your wrist as mentioned above and count the number of "pulses" that occur in fifteen seconds. Multiply that figure by four to determine your pulse rate per minute.

Training Heart Rate

Your maximum heart rate (per minute) can be determined by subtracting your age in years from 220. Your most effective "training heart rate" is determined by multiplying your maximum heart rate by 0.65 to 0.80. These values give you the desired range for your heart rate to reach and maintain during exercise.

Calculating training heart rate:

For example: Let us assume that you are 45 years old

220 minus 45 = 175

your maximum heart rate per minute

175 times 0.65/0.80 = 114 to 140

your training heart rate range per minute

To raise your heart rate to a desired level of aerobic benefit, you should maintain your level of exercise for a period of 20 minutes or longer. If you are taking your pulse for 15 seconds, divide your training heart rate by 4 since there are four 15 second intervals in one minute (for example 140 divided by 4 = 35 pulses) to give you a projected target rate in a 15 second interval. It is simpler and easier to take your pulse rate for 15 instead of 60 seconds. Once you get used to exercising, you will be able to "feel" when you reach your training heart rate. You may then need to only check your heart rate sporadically.

The downside of all this is that as you get leaner and lighter, it will take less energy to move your body. Less energy expended equals fewer calories burned. Therefore, you will need to work harder to burn the same number of calories you burned as you began your exercise program. Granted, this does not seem fair, but it is the truth. Try to maintain a positive attitude about the new "leaner" you, and keep exercising.

Learning to Enjoy Exercise

I sincerely believe that you will learn to enjoy exercise once you realize it is your body's friend. One of my clients, who I had a very hard time convincing to exercise, found that walking briskly was not as hard and boring as she expected. In fact, she ended up considering it a wonderful experience. She now glows with a sense of well-being and is very excited to be melting down her body fat after many years of failed attempts.

Exercise helps us in other ways, too. For example, exercise can also help reduce high blood pressure and lower a cholesterol count. It is the best thing you can do to increase your HDL, the good fat that helps our body remove excess cholesterol. Regular exercise can reduce your risk for heart attack or stroke; it can improve sleep, and it can normalize bowel function.

When you are stressed, exercise is wonderful. If I have not exercised for a period of time, because of traveling or unexpected responsibilities, I can always feel my body tension increase. Since I am a very disciplined person, this then compounds my stress levels. I try to make time in my daily routine (no matter how pressing) to include some exercise, even if I can only do a few minutes. This effort helps me relax and rejuvenates me. I find I can also think more clearly and solve problems while I'm exercising.

You may also experience a "clearing" of your mind. Perhaps this experience will afford you some time to slow down and "smell the roses" or "enjoy the sunshine." I may sound like I'm trying to sell you stock in an exercise studio, but I assure you I'm not. I know the multiple benefits of regular exercise and its availability to anyone and everyone, regardless of age, budget, or time. Exercise will also enhance your self-esteem and self-confidence;

you will experience a greater sense of satisfaction as you see yourself accomplishing your goals. What's not to love about such a great overall life enhancer!

Thirty Minutes a Day

My general recommendation is to exercise for a *minimum* of thirty minutes daily. This should create a "need" in your body to burn 250 calories per day, which will enhance your fat loss efforts and improve your cardiovascular fitness at the same time. If you should miss a day for whatever reason, don't fall into old patterns of "throwing the baby out with the bath water". Don't go back into the bondage of that old pattern of thinking that you just can't follow through with anything. Tell yourself that *tomorrow* is a brand new opportunity to get on with it. Do not wait until "the first of the week", "after the weekend", "Saturday morning", or whatever your body usually tries to "tell" you to do. Just determine to jump out of bed and start right back into your training mode again.

Exercise will help to replace the undesired excess fat tissue in your body with an increased amount of muscle tissue. No, not body-bulking muscles, but the desirable body muscle tissue that gives you the firm, toned, lean body you have always wanted.

Now, remember that a pound of pure muscle tissue is 80% water, while fat tissue is only 15% water.

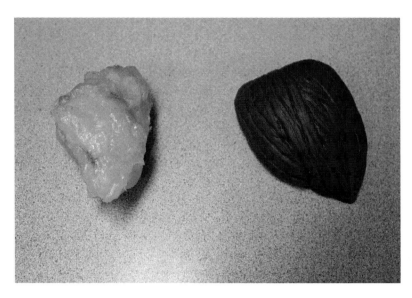

1 lb. FAT	1 lb. MUSCLE
15% water	80% water
3, 500 calories	400 calories

When you first start exercising, the scale numbers may stubbornly refuse to budge. They may even go *up*. This is related to your body shifting its fluid (water) balance. As this shifting of body fluid goes on, you will find that you feel "thinner" on the inside; your clothes are fitting differently, yet your longtime "enemy" the scale may not change much at all. *Do not worry!* You will be losing *fat* and that's what this is all about.

Another helpful side effect of aerobic exercise is that it usually decreases appetite. This is opposite of what we have sometimes heard, isn't it? Some of you may find that you are never hungry. This is really exciting if your whole life has previously revolved around feeling hungry all the time. When you eat less, your body wants to slow down in response to less fuel. Your exercise program prevents this from happening.

You can lose weight (fat) without starving!

Another positive side of exercising is that there are a wide variety of activities that you can pursue. If you are really creative, you might chase butterflies around a meadow, climb the pyramids in Egypt, square dance with an energetic partner every day, or perhaps wrestle longhorn cattle, just as long as your heart rate is *elevated* and *sustained* for thirty minutes or more. If more traditional examples appeal to you, try walking, biking, swimming, jogging, hiking, rowing machine, exercise bicycle, etc. Or, alternate ice-skating and skiing with swimming and biking. Develop a variety of indoor as well as outdoor activities you can do. Remember you need exercise all year, even if it's foggy and raining outside.

A pair of good cross-training shoes is important no matter whether you're walking, running, cycling, or hiking. Clothing should be comfortable and layered for weather conditions. You will be happy to know that you do *not* have to purchase expensive exercise equipment or pricey exercise clothes to be effective. You can, if you want to; you just don't have to!

We can also utilize technology to enhance our exercise efforts. We can watch virtual exercise programs while on a variety of exercise equipment. There are also electronic games that allow you to compete with others indoors using the television or computer. This can be fun, as well as exercise. Applications can be downloaded onto mobile devices and computers to track any number of activities. A novel use of GPS (global positioning system) is geocaching. This is a form of a scavenger hunt using the GPS settings to find clues.

If you are an individual who likes group activities, then sports teams like basketball, softball, hockey, football, etc. may be a good choice for you. Remember the time you spend with your heart rate consistently elevated is important. For example, if you are an outfielder in baseball you can keep moving in place while waiting for a ball to come your way.

Body Shaping and Toning

In addition to aerobic exercise, the following are examples of stretching and toning exercises that will help you shape up and achieve certain body-shaping goals.   Always remember to drink plenty of fluids—8 to 10 glasses per day of water, coffee, tea, or other non-caloric liquids. The total volume of fluid required is satisfied when the urine is dilute or very pale in color. This is very important for maintaining the resiliency of your skin. Your age, genetics, and the degree of your weight problem influence how your skin will look as you lose weight. Only in extreme cases is it necessary to contemplate cosmetic surgery to remove excess skin. This is a serious decision that should not be considered until your desired weight loss has been maintained for a minimum of six months.

1. To warm up, stand with your feet apart, arms hanging down with your palms resting against your side. Raise your arms over your head. Then lower your left elbow to meet your raised right knee. Resume your original position. Repeat with your right elbow lowering to meet your raised left knee. Repeat 20 times.

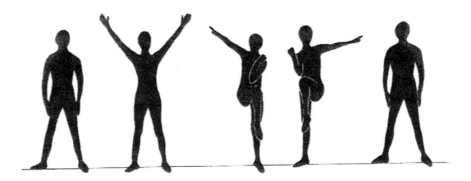

2. For hips and buttocks, kneel on your hands and knees and lower your head until it rests on your hands. Keep the palms of your hands flat on the floor and your back straight. First raise your right leg, with your

knee bent, until your upper leg (thigh) is in a straight line with your buttocks. Return to starting position. Repeat with left leg. Gradually increase number of repetitions until you do 20 lifts with each leg.

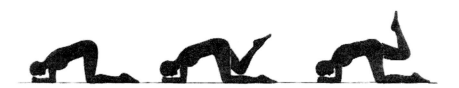

3.   For upper arms and torso, lie flat on the floor on your stomach with your palms flat on the floor at your shoulder level. Slowly lift upper body while knees remain on the floor. Gradually increase to 20 push-ups (from knees if you are female).

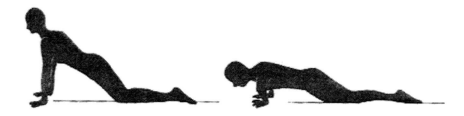

4.   For legs and inner thighs, stand with your feet apart and toes pointed out. Hold your arms straight out from your body at shoulder level. Slowly bend your knees, lowering your body as far as possible, keeping your buttocks directly above your feet. Gradually increase to 20 bends.

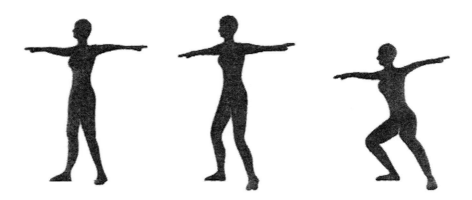

5. For your waist, stand with your feet apart and pointed forward. Your knees should be slightly bent. Raise and curl your left arm across your head in a half circle, keeping your right arm at waist level. With a circular motion, reverse your arms' position. You should feel a pull at your waist. Gradually increase this left-right reversal to 20 repetitions.

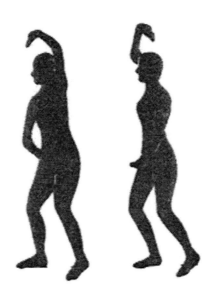

6.   For your stomach, lie on your back on the floor. Bend your knees and cross your arms over your chest. Keep your back as flat to the floor as you can. Slowly raise your head and shoulders just off the floor, and hold that position for a count of 5 (five seconds). Then slowly lower your upper body back to the floor. Gradually increase to 20 repetitions. When done properly, this exercise will strengthen abdominal muscles while not straining your back.

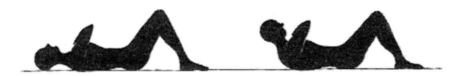

Resistance Training

Resistance or strength training has been demonstrated to reverse the loss of lean muscle mass and bone as we age. After age forty, the sedentary amongst us can lose from 20 to 40% of their muscle mass. Unfortunately, this makes it easier to gain weight.

Weight or strength training should be done three times a week. For your upper body you will need three to eight lb. weights and five to twelve lb. weights for the lower body. You can determine the appropriate weight with practice. You need to do

8 to 12 repetitions to challenge your muscles. If it is too easy to complete the 12 reps, choose a heavier weight and vice versa. The amount of weight should be just enough to provide resistance, but not so much to make it too difficult; you may increase the number of reps if you like.

Start with the large muscles in your hips and legs. Then move to your back, followed by your chest and arms. Last you will work your abdominal or stomach muscles.

1. Lunge. With legs two to three feet apart and weights in each hand, bend front leg while keeping back straight; repeat with other leg.

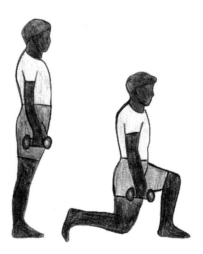

2. Back Lateral. While seated, lean slightly forward. Raise your arms up and back, bringing weights to shoulder level.

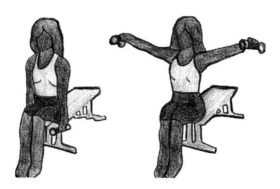

3. Bent Row. Lean on stool. With other hand, lift weight by pulling arm up; lift elbow high. Repeat with both arms.

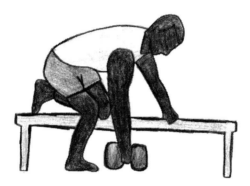

4. Flies. With arms straight out, elbows slightly bent, bring weights across chest.

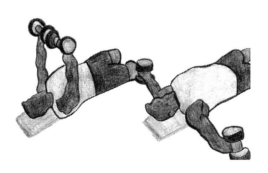

5. Side Laterals. Raise weights outward to shoulder level.

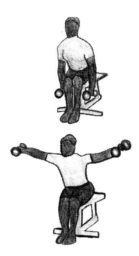

6. Alternating Press. While seated or standing, lift one arm with weight above head; return. Repeat with both arms.

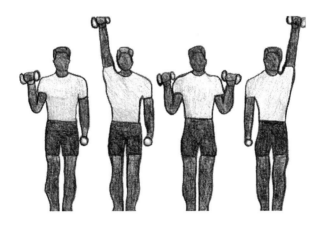

7. Curls. Lift one weight to chest; return. Lift the opposite weight.

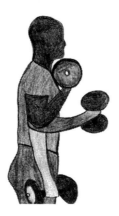

Weight/Carbohydrate/Exercise Graph

The graph on the following page will help you track your weight, exercise, and food in a very visual way. The graph includes thirty-one columns across the top. Each column represents one day in a month. In each column there will be a maximum of three types of information recorded. A "·" representing weight, an "X" representing carbohydrate intake, and squares of color representing minutes of exercise completed for that day.

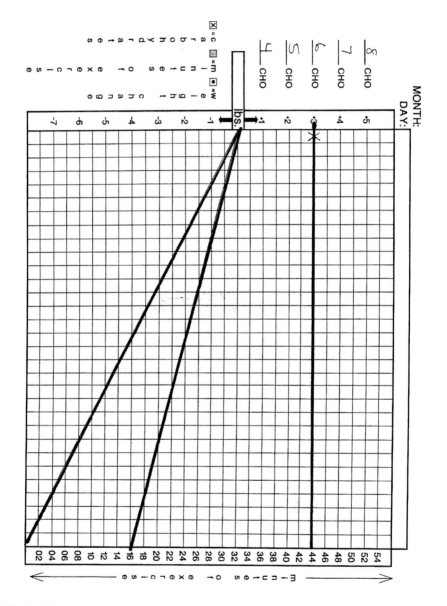

Weight/Carbohydrate/Exercise Graph

Weight

You may weigh daily or weekly. Your weight should always be measured at the same time of day, and you should be dressed (or undressed) in the same fashion each time. Most people prefer to weigh first thing in the morning without clothing (we generally weigh the least then).

When recording your weight on the graph, you will use a "·" to symbolize your weight. Your starting weight is placed on the "0" line in the first column. The numbers in the column on the left side of the graph refer to pounds of weight change. Each square is valued at 1/2 pound. For example, if your current or starting weight is 200, then at −1, you would put 199 (200 minus 1 = 199); at −2, you would put 198 (200 minus 2 = 198) and so on. Since your goal is to lose between 4 to 8 pounds a month, you can insert goal lines for the month. These diagonal target lines are drawn from the zero line on the left to the −4 on the right and from the zero line on the left to the −8 on the right as shown on the example.

You will place a weight "·" in one column each day of the month (if you are weighing daily). As you track the differences in your weight (daily or weekly), you will be able to see how close you are to your monthly target goals. Once you have the dots across the graph, you may connect them. The slope of this line will give you feedback on how you are doing as the month progresses. You can compare your progress to the target lines you inserted earlier.

Exercise

Minutes of exercise are noted in the extreme right hand column of the graph. Each square is valued at 2 minutes, increasing as you go up the graph. Use a felt-tip pen or color pencil to make a bar graph, which reflects the number of minutes you exercise each day. For each day or column, color in the number of squares, that represent the number of minutes of exercise for that day. Your goal is to have the lower part of this graph solidly colored in. If you miss exercise for several days, you have immediate feedback when the area is not colored in. You will also see the relationship in how your weight loss is affected. When you exercise regularly, your weight loss will be better.

If you would like to modify the chart to reflect steps per day, count every 2 squares as 1,000 steps (instead of minutes) starting from the bottom and going up the right-hand side. Your goal of 10,000 steps will coincide with 40 minutes. The purpose of a pedometer is to track all the steps you take during a day. It can be very motivating for both adults and children. A simple and easy to use pedometer is Model SW-200 from New-Lifestyles. It does not require any calibrating. Each day you open it up and push one button to re-set the number of steps to zero. This is worn at the waist and I suggest securing it with a safety strap as well, since pedometers tend to pop off and get lost or broken.

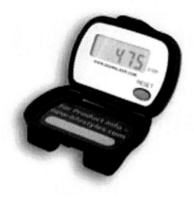

Carbohydrate

The third component of the graph is the way you will track your eating plan or behavior.

Your eating plan has several fixed or controlled components.

1. An assigned number of ounces of high quality protein per day.

2. A minimum of four servings of vegetables per day.

3. A low fat intake per day (goal of 30% or fewer total calories from fat).

Given the above, the number of carbohydrate servings in your plan is what is recorded on the graph to give you feedback on your weight loss progress. The number of servings can be adjusted to control your rate of fat/weight loss.

To simplify the process, we will categorize the amount of carbohydrate in your plan as carbohydrate servings (CHOs). A CHO (carbohydrate serving) is a food which provides primarily carbohydrate calories at 15 grams/ serving. When you refer back to the Food Guide information, you will see that both fruit and bread/cereal groups provide 15 grams carbohydrate per serving.

Examples of CHOs are:

½ cup fruit or juice

1 slice or 1 oz. bread

½ cup potato, corn, cooked dry beans

1/3 cup pasta or rice

1 oz. cereal by weight

Since one cup of nonfat milk contains 12 grams carbohydrate and 8 grams of protein, it counts two ways: as a CHO (carbohydrate) serving and a PRO (protein) serving; this same rule also applies to legumes, such as cooked dry beans. On the top section of the graph in the left margin area, you will designate a range of CHO servings. For example, your basic plan includes six servings. On the graph, you will track a range from four to eight servings, with each line being worth 1/2 serving. You will place an "X" over the line that represents the number of CHO (carbohydrate) servings you consumed on that day. You might include a bold line of color at level 6 as your target CHO intake. As the month progresses, you can easily see how closely you are following your plan by how far the X's are moving from your target line.

Your "discretionary calories" are also assigned as CHO choices. This is an arbitrary designation and does *not* mean that the calories of all CHO choices are the same. For example, 1 oz. chocolate has more fat than 1/2 cup fruit, but the CHO content is approximately the same. When you choose a variety of CHO choices, including those high in fat and sugar, this simplified system allows you to eat the foods you enjoy. Let's say you are in a "choco-late" mood; this system would allow you to have as much as 6 oz. chocolate (6 CHO) for the day, and still fall within the guidelines of your target plan. Granted, this extreme in choices is not the "variety" we want in the long run, but it allows you the flexibility of eating those foods you like.

Our job is to determine the best CHO level for you. When you eat a lot of extra CHO servings, you will see that your weight goes up quickly because of the metabolic water, which is produced as these foods are digested. Unfortunately, it can take up to seven days for this water to go away again. When you know these facts, it is easier to understand that quick fluctuations in weight are *not* related to fat loss. It is critical that you continue your positive changes in behavior, and not let the scale control your behavior. What is important is the change on the scale over time, not the day-to-day changes.

FALLACY #1:

"I'm *good* if the scale goes down."

FALLACY #2:

"I can't do *anything* right if the scale goes up."

TRUTH #1:

"I'm good if I exercise thirty minutes a day."

TRUTH #2:

"I'm doing well when I follow my meal plan the best I can."

Chapter 10

Positive Mental Programming

In this day and age it seems that we are constantly on the run. We have little time for ourselves, especially if we are raising a family and work outside the home. There is even less time for rest and relaxation, resulting in stress. Living in a constant state of stress inevitably produces frustration and wrong reactions. What wrong reactions are you aware of in your life? Is one of your reactions to the stresses of everyday living, to eat? Are you using food to reward yourself, to reduce anxiety, to cheer yourself up, to please someone else, to alleviate boredom, to dissipate anger, to be happy, and other wrong reasons for eating? These are examples of behavioral issues we will discuss in a later chapter.

Positive mental programming is a simple tool you can learn to help you cope with a variety of issues. I use this mental technique when I am going to give a lecture or talk. Some time ago I was asked to take the place of a major speaker at a physicians' meeting. With only thirty minutes' notice, I had to convince myself that my talk, which had originally been prepared for nursing staff, could be delivered positively and confidently to such an audience. I spent twenty-five of those minutes telling myself over and over that I would do the best I possibly could, that I would smile, that I would not talk too fast, that I would not fill pauses with "ahs" and "you knows." I really had a good feeling when I finished speaking, and the feedback from the audience was positive as well.

Positive mental programming is a skill that you can learn and will want to practice daily. This ability to tune out the world is like daydreaming; we all go in and out of this state many times a day without even realizing it. It is similar to meditation. In your case, I want you to focus your attention on controlling your eating habits.

You, and you alone, are able to take control of your own thoughts. You will not do anything when you are deeply relaxed that you would not consciously allow. No one can make you do anything you do not want to do yourself. Once you read this chapter, you may want to make a recording of the process to easily learn the technique. As you gain experience in this mental reinforcement technique, you will be able to relax more quickly and efficiently. Eventually, you will not desire or need to use a recording.

For example, let's suppose you have been invited to someone's home for dinner. You are now going to use your imagination to create mental pictures about this upcoming dinner. You can "practice" being at the dinner by using your imagination. Imagine as much detail as possible to help your images be more realistic. See yourself mingling with the other guests, rather than "standing guard" at the hors d'oeuvres table. When you are at the dinner table, picture yourself taking small bites and chewing everything well. Imagine being satisfied with a small amount of everything, feeling no compulsion or need to "clean" your plate.

You will have a small serving of dessert, if you like, since you have planned that as part of your discretionary calories for the day. As you are enjoying the fine meal your host and hostess have prepared for you, concentrate on an imaginary discussion of several lively topics going on around the table. Tell yourself that you do not feel deprived and you are in control.

To practice this imagery, you need to find a time and place that will allow you about twenty minutes of uninterrupted quiet. You will find it helpful to relax in the same place at the same time every day. Get as comfortable as you can, relaxing in a favorite recliner or even lying down if you prefer. Your clothing should be loose and comfortable, and you may want to cover yourself with a light blanket. If you wear glasses or contact lenses, remove them before starting to relax since you need to close your eyes.

Script for Positive Mental Programming

When you are comfortable in your relaxing position, take a deep breath and exhale. Then point your toes and stretch your legs as far as they can go, tighten the muscles in your feet and hold them for several seconds. Next, tighten the muscles in your calves and those in your thighs. As you make your entire leg as tight as you can, inhale and hold your breath. Hold it some more. Then let your breath out, and let go of every muscle you're aware of in your lower body. Relax all the muscles in your toes, all the muscles in your calves, all the muscles in your thighs. Let your legs go completely limp. Expect to feel a wonderful relaxation coming up from your toes, up your calves, up your thighs. Expect to begin to feel wonderfully relaxed and calm.

Stretch out your fingers. Curl them in and make a tight fist. Think about how the tightness feels. Clench your fists tighter, as tightly as you can, and hold them in that state. Tighten the muscles in your wrists, in your forearms, in your upper arms. Hold them in that state while you inhale deeply. Hold that breath, then exhale and begin to relax. Let yourself relax all over, and notice the feeling of relaxation going through your fingers, your hands, your forearms, and now your upper arms. Let your arms go completely limp. Expect to begin feeling very relaxed, very comfortable, and very calm.

Now arch your back, raising your chest upward. Tighten your neck and shoulder muscles, tighten your stomach muscles, but continue to breathe regularly. Make all those muscles as tight as you can, make them tighter and tighter, and hold them in that state. Finally, begin to let go; just let every muscle go. Expect to feel completely relaxed. Feel the muscles relaxing from your back, from your shoulders, from your chest, from your stomach.

Now tighten the muscles in your face. You may make a funny face. Tighten the muscles around your mouth, the muscles in your chin, around your eyes and your forehead. Wrinkle your eyebrows. Make them tighter and tighter, and hold it for several seconds. Then let go. Notice how relaxed the muscles are in your forehead, the muscles around your eyes, the muscles in your cheeks, the muscles in your chin, and the muscles around your mouth. Expect to feel wonderfully relaxed and very calm.

At this point, take a very deep breath and hold it gently but as long as you can. Now slowly let it out. With it go all your tensions, your frustrations, and your anxieties. Be aware of how relaxed you are feeling.

Now we will proceed to "mentally" relax every part of your body progressively. You will be aware of your surroundings, although you may care less and less about what goes on around you. Direct your thoughts to the top of your head, and notice that whatever tension exists there, is rapidly vanishing. Your scalp is becoming less and less tight, and the top of your head is becoming completely relaxed. And now think of your forehead, and let all the muscles in your forehead relax and become loose and limp. And now your eyes, and all the small muscle groups around your eyes. Just allow them to become loose and limp and relaxed. Relax more and more, and let yourself go completely. Now relax your facial muscles, the muscles in your cheeks and around your nose, and the muscles around your mouth and teeth. Just let them all relax and let them all go very loose and limp.

Now relax the muscles in your throat area, and let them all relax. Now think of your shoulders, and permit your shoulder muscles to relax. Relax the muscles in your upper arms, your elbows, and your forearms; relax all the muscles up and down your arms. Just let them go loose and limp. Your wrists, your hands, your very fingers are completely relaxed.

Now relax all the muscles in your chest, the muscles in your stomach area, and your abdomen. Allow all your muscles to become very loose and limp. Now think of your back and all the muscles up and down your back; let all these muscles relax completely.

Now think of your thighs and relax all of those muscles, the muscles in your knees, and the muscles in your calves. And just let all of those muscles relax completely-your ankles, your feet, and your toes. Relax and let go completely.

Regardless of your past experiences with losing weight, you are now beginning a new program of constructive and helpful suggestions. Now, as you continue to work on relaxing every day, you will begin to realize that you can change your wrong eating habits. You will practice new healthy eating habits, and you will maintain your weight once you have reached your goal. You will realize that as you see yourself more positively, you will be more determined to reach your goals. Your self esteem will improve daily. You will be able to control your healthy food choices and maintain an attractive and healthy body. You will be more and more determined every day.

Now, when you are tempted to eat out of control, your new self-image and increasing sense of well being will cause you to ask yourself: "Do I really want to do this? Won't I feel better if I exercise control and notice how satisfied I can be with just a small amount? Since I can eat the foods I enjoy, I do not feel that I am on a restrictive diet."

Now, I want you to get a clear mental picture of how you wish to look when you have attained your goal. See yourself at your goal weight. Visualize yourself wearing an attractive dress or suit. Get a clear mental picture of your new slim self-image. Now look at yourself very closely. Notice how well you look with your stomach flat; how firm your face looks without the extra chin. Look at the smooth profile you have with your slimmer hips. Each time you enter this relaxed state, this image will become clearer and more lifelike. Notice and experience the feeling of happiness arising within you, along with a rising sense of confidence that your goal can be reached. Once you feel this in your present, relaxed state of mind, you will soon begin to think of yourself in this manner during your ordinary waking hours.

Whenever you are tempted to eat out of control or whenever your positive mental attitude starts to slip, all you need to do is to use a "signal", such as looking at a picture of yourself at your goal weight, or whatever signal you decide to use. When you use that signal, you will quickly get a mental picture of your new self-image. You will be able to reproduce this feeling of happiness and determination that you can do it. The amount of pleasure that you will derive knowing that you can lose weight will be so great that the temporary gratification of your taste buds will seem small in comparison.

Now, see yourself as a trim and attractive person at a pleasant social gathering. Notice friends congratulating you on your new appearance. Notice how much energy you have, and see the envy in the eyes of all your friends who are still overweight. Now watch yourself eating. See yourself taking smaller portions, enjoying the subtle flavor of the food, and eating more slowly to savor every bite. Imagine being so satisfied that you can even leave something on your plate. See yourself refusing second helpings because you already feel so full. You feel a great sense of accomplishment in saying "no" to more.

And now, just enjoy the wonderful feeling of relaxation. You are feeling calm and relaxed; you feel completely calm and at ease. You will practice this deep state of relaxation and give yourself positive suggestions regularly. You will see mental pictures of yourself reacting positively in any situation.

Now that you are feeling so good and so full of self-confidence, I am going to ask you to rouse yourself. When you do, you will feel refreshed, alert, and completely comfortable. Each time you enter this state, you will be able to relax more rapidly and deeply. All the suggestions you give yourself will assist you in reaching your goals, and you will feel better than you have in a long time. Every day you will gain more confidence in your ability to succeed in managing your weight control program. Now, blink your eyes to open them, and notice how good you feel.

Chapter 11

What Are Your Behavior Patterns?

Have you ever been hungry? Are you sure? Many of my overweight patients realize that they do *not* know what it actually means to be *physiologically hungry*. Many people have learned to eat in response to situations such as a particular place, an event, or with a particular person. Others might eat in response to emotions or feelings—such as anger, frustration, loneliness, and boredom.

> **In general, the person with a weight problem eats in response to external or emotional cues rather than internal hunger.**

Because you may have learned to respond to external or emotional cues to eat, rather than internal hunger, let's look at your behavior patterns to learn how you are influenced to eat. We'll find out what cues are you responding to when you think you are feeling hungry. To do this, you first need to write down everything you normally eat during a typical day in your life. You will also need to write down where you eat each item, and how you feel as you are eating the item. Do not try to change your present eating habits for this exercise. We need a true picture of where you are right now with your food cues. Keep this detailed list for three days total, *including one weekend day.*

Here are three Daily Journal pages for you to record your meals. As you move across the top of the page, you need to also carefully note the time of the day or evening that you are eating. Down the left side of the form are various notes you need to make.

1. Write down what you are eating.

2. Note how many minutes it takes you to eat.

3. Note the location where you are eating, bedroom, living room, etc.

4. Note your position: walking, standing, sitting, etc.

5. Note what you are doing while you are eating.

6. Note who are you with: family members, friend, alone, etc.

7. Note what your mood is: angry, depressed, frustrated, etc.

8. Note how hungry you are: 0 = not hungry, 5 = very hungry, or a number in between.

9. Note any exercise or activity in minutes.

Day 1 Daily Journal

	Breakfast	Lunch	Dinner	Snacks
Time of day				
Quantity/food				
Time spent eating				
Location				
Position				
Doing what				
With whom				
Mood				
Degree hunger				
Activity				
Remarks/observations:				

Day 2 Daily Journal

	Breakfast	Lunch	Dinner	Snacks
Time of day				
Quantity/food				
Time spent eating				
Location				
Position				
Doing what				
With whom				
Mood				
Degree hunger				
Activity				
Remarks/observations:				

	Breakfast	Lunch	Dinner	Snacks
Day 3 Daily Journal				
Time of day				
Quantity/food				
Time spent eating				
Location				
Position				
Doing what				
With whom				
Mood				
Degree hunger				
Activity				
Remarks/observations:				

What do you feel you can learn from keeping this daily journal? I hope you see it as a source of new information, facts that you may not have recognized earlier. The journal becomes the basis of identifying behavior pattern areas you will want to change. Do *not* make the mistake of trying to change everything all at once. I would suggest that you identify the easiest things to change and do them first. This will give you a sense of accomplishment and satisfaction. Then gradually work toward the areas that are harder for you to change.

Examples of Problem Behaviors

Problem #1: Starve and Stuff

The time of day may be a problem for you if you do not eat anything all day long, and then seem to be unable to stop eating from the moment you get home in the evening. Your body will use your calories more effectively and you will be less hungry if you eat smaller meals throughout the day. You may argue that if you eat in the morning, then you're hungry all day. This will certainly be so if you eat mostly sources of sugar such as doughnuts, muffins or sweet rolls. Remember, the ingredients of these sources of calories turn into almost all sugar that will result in a sharp rise and subsequent fall in your blood sugar. This is a "red alert" to your body that you are *hungry*.

A Possible Solution:

Combine adequate high quality protein *with* the carbo-hydrate you eat. This will help you be more satisfied and less hungry. For example, choose 1 oz. low fat cheese on one slice of whole grain bread.

Problem # 2: When to Say "When"

Your problem may simply be too--large portions of every-thing. Most of the time, the excessive portions are in the area of hidden fat and sugar, such as cheese, nuts or snack foods. I've never seen anyone eat too many veg-etables!

A Possible Solution:

Use smaller plates and containers for your servings. Mea-sure your portions of everything you will be eating before sitting down to dine. Try not to prepare more than the portion recommended in your menu pattern, but if you do prepare larger amounts for convenience' sake, imme-diately place the leftover food into containers, and put it in the refrigerator before sitting down to eat.

Problem #3: Food Inhaler

How fast you eat is a very important factor in your eating program. If you are eating a meal in less than five to ten minutes, barely pausing between bites, it will be easy for you to eat too much. It takes your stomach about twenty minutes to "register fullness" by sending a signal to your brain that you've had enough to eat. So, if the only cue that you recognize to stop eating is when you finally feel "satisfied", you are probably overeating. This is especially true in direct relationship to how fast you eat. You will end up feeling stuffed, way past true satisfaction, and you will feel uncomfortable afterward as well.

A Possible Solution:

Slow down your rate of eating. Concentrate on chewing each mouthful well. Put down your silverware between bites, perhaps conversing with those at the table, etc. If you are dining alone, pause between bites and contemplate a leaner you and all the things you will want to do with your new body. If you have learned to eat quickly, it may seem difficult at first to slow down and change your eating behavior. But practice, practice, practice, and you will succeed.

Problem #4: Mindless Munching

Where you eat may influence your pattern of eating. For example, you may be used to eating in front of the television, perhaps even so "programmed" that you rarely eat without the television as your meal partner. Concentrating on what your "meal partners" are saying, you may be totally unaware of *what* and how *much* you are actually putting into your mouth. For example, it is easy to sit down with a box of crackers and a beverage and mindlessly munch away. When we do this, we rarely pay attention to how many crackers we are eating-- we just reach in and grab a few, again and again and again. By the end of the evening, we may have consumed the whole box, just a little bit at a time.

In addition to this "mindless" eating while distracted with your electronic "companion", you may be influenced by, and even given subconscious suggestions by, commercials to want to eat a variety of "caloric and fatty foods". Even if you did not sit down with the crackers, you may be triggered to go out to get something you saw advertised to eat.

A Possible Solution:

Establish a designated eating place in your home that is away from the television and any other distraction. This way you can determine what and how much you are going to eat. For example, set out on a plate six crackers and 1 oz. of low fat cheese with a beverage. Eat these foods slowly, pausing to enjoy the various flavors and textures. Then, when you are finished, move to the other room to watch television.

Problem #5: The Kitchen Disposal

Do you grab something to eat the moment you hit the kitchen? Or every time you walk by the refrigerator? This is a very common habit, and the pattern is helped by having easy-to-eat foods in easy reach on the counters or in plain sight in the refrigerator. Unless you are determined to pay attention to everything you put in your mouth, it is easy to snack this way all day long. You may then find that you are not particularly hungry at dinner time, so to make up for your earlier snacking, you decide it would be best to just skip eating with the family. This is a mistake, for you will almost always resume the snacking pattern later in the evening.

You may truly be at a loss as to why you can't seem to lose weight since you feel that you do not even eat every meal of the day---no dinner Tuesday night, no lunch Wednesday, no breakfast Thursday. How can anyone keep gaining weight on such a pattern of deprivation, right? Since you are usually grabbing foods high in simple sugar and fat as you snack or mindlessly munch between the missed meals, weight gain is inevitable.

A Possible Solution:

Put all the foods that you grab mindlessly out of sight, preferably in a deep cupboard and out of easy reach. As funny as this might sound, you could try something as creative or dramatic as wearing a surgical-type mask while in the kitchen. This extra step, silly or not, will help you be aware of and break the automatic cycle of putting things in your mouth when you are not focused on what you are doing.

Problem #6: The Eat-and-Run Eater

We have all had to eat on the run sometimes—it is a curse of the hectic lifestyle of the age we live in. But we can also be sure to plan ahead for adequate eating, if we choose to believe that this is as important a habit as brushing our teeth or combing our hair.

A Possible Solution:

Eating only when sitting down may help you break this pattern. For example, if you are a "commuter" and drive your car every day, you may frequently eat fast food. You may need to decide to never eat in your car. This might entail getting up a littler earlier to eat properly before you leave home in the morning, or, you may be able to eat while commuting as long as you prepare appropriate foods that you can transport with you.

For example, when I commuted an hour each way to my office, I would pack my breakfast meal the night before. I could then enjoy a leisurely meal on the way to the office rather than trying to eat quickly before I headed out the door.

Problem #7: The Food Monitor/Food Pusher

Who you are *with* may also affect what and how much you eat. You may have someone who is monitoring your food intake. When they see you eating something they feel is inappropriate, they may comment to you. In this circumstance, they are "parenting" you. Unless you are in complete control of which *inner you* (your adult, your parent, or your child) is currently handling your reactions, your typical response may well be to eat even more in rebellion or defiance, much like a child who is being reprimanded. You then become enmeshed in a power struggle over food. The opposite situation may occur when the person you are with has one or more of the behavior patterns described here or encourages you to eat *more* than you really want.

A Possible Solution:

Whether you are alone or with someone else, you need to be honest with yourself about what and how much you eat. As an adult you have a right to eat what you want. It is <u>extremely </u>important for you to learn that there are no forbidden foods, no good foods/bad foods. You can choose to include whatever you want to eat in a well-balanced eating pattern that will work for you. Since your needs are different from day to day, some days you may be really hungry, and you may need to eat more. Some days a piece of chocolate candy is exactly what you want. It is okay for you to eat that piece of chocolate candy as long as it is a "reasonable" amount.

Don't go back into self-defeating behavior or self-talk that may sound something like this: "Eating that piece of chocolate candy is 'off' my diet, so I've blown the whole program. Well! I might as well just eat the rest of the box since I've gone this far. I'll start my diet again on Monday."

Many of the behavioral aspects of your eating will be reflected in your moods. You may eat when happy or sad, tired or frustrated, angry or depressed, or when bored or stressed. The first step is to recognize what influences you, then work to substitute positive behavior to the response of wanting to eat if you're in a negative mood and not hungry.

If your charts and journals have shown you that you have been eating when you weren't truly hungry, you need to get in tune with your body's hunger signals. You need to first learn to recognize what true physiological hunger feels like. Some people might have to wait for twelve to eighteen hours before they identify true hunger pangs. This is because we have a tendency to stuff ourselves so much that our bodies have given up trying to signal us that it is time to give it more food.

Test yourself by trying to wait for your next meal until you are truly physiologically hungry. Some people become so programmed by the clock that hearing a clock chime noon causes them to begin salivating just like Pavlov's dogs did when the bell rang. "Lunchtime, gonna get to eat, oh boy, oh boy, lunchtime." My father could eat a huge breakfast, but still want lunch exactly at noon. He was used to eating by the clock, not his stomach.

If you are really hungry, your stomach will "growl." These sounds will actually dissipate if ignored, only to reappear some time later. This is a true physiological signal that it is time to provide nourishment for your body. Your appetite, on the other hand, is just the desire to eat. You may feel that you really want to eat, and the feeling does not go away. This is a desire rather than a *need* to eat. You literally "think" you are hungry.

Try to concentrate on eating only when you are actually hungry. Your use of the Daily Journal should help you identify areas that may be a problem for you. If you begin to feel overwhelmed by the process and the many areas on which you need to work, remember that you did not learn all these bad habits at once, and you probably won't unlearn them all at once, either. So, lighten up on yourself if you're feeling overwhelmed. You will be successful by tackling them one at a time.

It can take six months to learn a new habit. For example, thinking about writing this book seemed like an overwhelming task to contemplate, let alone consider completing. When I divided the material into smaller sections, then the whole book became more manageable. As sections were completed, I realized how much progress I was making on the overall project.

Four Questions

Another helpful technique to determine if your hunger is real or false, or simply a craving, is to ask yourself these four questions.

1. Am I really hungry?

Look back over the suggestions I've enumerated above to help you discern the answer to this question.

2. What specifically do I want to eat?

If you really want chocolate, do not try to substitute something else. Typically, in trying to resist a strong food desire, you may start out to eat something else, but nothing satisfies you until you actually eat what you wanted in the first place.

3. How do I feel as I am eating?

This is the most important question and one people tend to ignore. The objective here is to pay attention to the sensory aspects of the food (flavor, texture, temperature, aroma, etc.).

I will never forget how I felt eating a banana split years ago. It was exactly what I wanted, and I was very hungry. In fact, I had skipped my dinner to allow for the calories. But as I was eating, the flavors all blended together, and pretty soon it didn't taste like much but a very sweet and rich concoction. I started to feel sick to my stomach. I didn't even care for bananas especially, so despite the longing that I had for such a "treat", it turned out to be very disappointing. I could not finish it.

4. Am I full?

If so, stop eating regardless of what is left in your bowl or on your plate. I left the highly-desired banana split, and I've never had the desire to have another one since. Actually, I prefer to order a small single-flavor sundae when I want a special treat. I have learned to be satisfied with a small amount of such a rich dessert.

Ask yourself these four questions the next time you feel hungry or "crave" a specific food.

Chapter 12

How to Change Your Behavioral Problems

Problem solving in our lives extends much further than just the area of weight loss. We need to solve problems of one variety or another every day of our lives. For example, suppose your family has one car and two members of the family need to be in different places at the same time. You need to work out a way to resolve the dilemma, perhaps arranging for the first person to be dropped off at the first location a little earlier so the second person is able to arrive at his destination on time.

I want to help you recognize effective problem-solving techniques that will help you be in control of your eating patterns. You have learned to eat with little or no control; now you need to eat while staying in control of your choices. You have probably learned to use food to cope with a variety of issues, most of them negative, and this caused you to form wrong habits. It would be nice if we could simply push a backspace or delete button and wipe out these old habits. Unfortunately, we can't. You will have to focus on first identifying what your old habits are, and then focus on changing them to more positive

habits. Each habit you change requires six months practice, or longer, before it becomes a steadfast new habit.

In the last chapter you identified your eating behaviors. The following pages summarize some of those eating problem areas once again. I recommend that you
select one habit, or two at the most, to concentrate on.
Start with the old habit that you think will be the easiest
to change.   Think of as many ways as possible for you
to solve the problem habit. Be as creative as you can
with multiple solutions. Then begin practicing the solution
or solutions.

Remember to set a realistic goal for resolving this first old
habit, not falling into the trap of setting a goal you can't
keep and then giving up entirely.

For example, suppose you have selected the problem:
"When to Say When". There are many ways you might
solve this problem area; the more creative you can be,
the more solutions you may be able to develop.

Possible solutions to help me know "when to say when":

1. Use smaller plates and containers.

2. Measure all portions.

3. Ask the Four Questions (Am I hungry? etc.)

4. Substitute another activity when bored: organize a closet or drawer, take a walk, etc.

5. Do a simple task that is not difficult: iron a skirt, water the lawn, walk the dog. Then when you go back to the problem that has frustrated you, the solution may come easily.

6. Do the task you have been putting off first during the day.

You may decide not to go grocery shopping when you are hungry. Your first goal may be not to shop when hungry for one week. If you succeed at this goal, then gradually extend it to a longer period of time. Before too long, shopping when you are not hungry will become your new habit pattern. Achieving small, manageable goals builds your confidence in your ability to succeed.

EATING PROBLEM AREAS

"Starve and Stuff"

I eat:

- snacks all day
- irregular meals
- on the run
- high sugar and high fat foods

"When to Say When"

I eat:

- when I am not hungry
- when I am bored
- when I am frustrated or procrastinating
- frequent second helpings
- large amounts of food

"Food Inhaler"

I eat:

- when I am angry
- when I am depressed
- when I am happy
- quickly; in fact I'm done in 5 to7 minutes

"Mindless Munching"

I eat:

- when I am clearing the table
- when I am eating out with others
- while I am cooking
- on my way home from the grocery store
- when I see something that looks good, even though I'm not hungry

- while reading, watching TV, or studying
- when driving the car

"Kitchen Disposal"

I eat:

- because there is something on my plate; I must clean my plate
- when the kids don't finish their meal
- when putting the groceries away after shopping
- as long as there is food in front of me

"Food Monitor/Food Pusher"

I eat:

- when someone says "you *must* have some, I made it just for you"
- when someone says "a little won't hurt; come on, join me!"
- more when someone is 'bugging' me; I will sneak food when no one is around

Be sure to add any other problems you have with eating.

On the pages that follow, list the problems you have identified above. Select one or two per week to work on. As you try the solutions you have decided might work, evaluate your performance. If the first solution you tried was less than successful, don't give up. Try another possibility until you find a solution that works well for you.

For example, if you use a smaller plate, but find yourself just piling your food higher and higher, that may not be a workable solution. However, if you continue to use a smaller plate, *and* measure all your food portions, that may work very well. Evaluate how well the solution seems to be working, and then choose to try it for another week, or choose to select another strategy.

When you move on to another problem area, try not to forget the area you have just worked to change. For example, suppose the first week your goal is not to shop when hungry. The second week you may move on to not eating in the car, but you find yourself shopping when hungry. This is a sign your are trying to change too much, too fast. Remember, be patient with yourself. You did not pick up all these negative behaviors in one or two weeks. You may need more time and practice to change. Just keep trying—over and over again.

Changing Bad Habits into Positive Solutions

Example for "Starve and Stuff"

Eating Habit	Possible Solution	My Self Evaluation
I snack all day	I will eat 3 meals and a planned evening snack.	I had 4 extra snacks this week. Next week I will have 2 extra snacks or less.

"Starve and Stuff"

Eating Habit	Possible Solution	My Self-Evaluation
1.		
2.		
3.		
4.		

"When to Say When"

Eating Habit	Possible Solution	My Self-Evaluation
1.		
2.		
3.		
4.		

"The Food Inhaler"

Eating Habit	Possible Solution	My Self-Evaluation
1.		
2.		
3.		
4.		

"Mindless Munching"

Eating Habit	Possible Solution	My Self-Evaluation
1.		
2.		
3.		
4.		

"Kitchen Disposal"

Eating Habit	Possible Solution	My Self-Evaluation
1.		
2.		
3.		
4.		

"Food Monitor/Food Pusher"

Eating Habit	Possible Solution	My Self-Evaluation
1.		
2.		
3.		
4.		

As you are planning to implement a change strategy, it may be helpful to mentally practice what you are going to do. This is applying what you learned earlier about visualization—in other words, you are going to "picture" yourself practicing the new behavior. Think positively about what you are doing; don't stress over making some mistakes. Making mistakes is just part of the overall process. Think about the toddler trying to learn how to walk—does he just get up and walk? No. Every little "walker" has practiced a variety of behaviors over a period of time. First he pulls himself around on all fours, then he pulls himself up on something. Gradually, he walks around a table before he strikes off across the floor.

Your long-term goals are to be balanced in body, mind, and lifestyle. Remember the E.A.T. Model. These questions may help you stay focused.

1.   Am I thinking positively?

2.   Are my expectations reasonable?

3.   Am I using words, not my weight, to express myself?

4.   Am I taking care of my body?

5.   Am I physically active?

6.   Do I take time to relax?

You will learn as you try new skills and solutions.

Persevere and you will succeed in your weight control process.

Chapter 13

What Do You Say to Yourself?

What you say to yourself silently is what I am going to call "self-talk." How you think, or talk to yourself, determines how you feel about yourself. For example, suppose you ate some popcorn at a movie. You might tell yourself, "I blew my whole diet; I can never lose weight; I can't do anything right". Listening to these negative thoughts in your own mind, without any editing of them or rejecting them, causes you to believe them. Believe them to be true, and it won't take long until you feel defeated. How you process these thoughts and how you can change them is the subject of this chapter.

Think back to an important point presented in Chapter 11—that true hunger is a physiological need and that in general:

A person with a weight problem generally eats in response to external or emotional cues rather than internal hunger.

Let's propose a hypothetical scenario: you are having a food problem starting from minor food ingestion, such as one cookie. Your "self-talk" might go something like this: "I'm on a 'diet', and I should not eat *any* cookies! It seems that I can't ever do anything right. I might as well just eat the rest of these stupid cookies, and then I won't have to worry about them." These negative thoughts immediately lead to negative feelings of failure, your failure, again.

The one bright spot here is the fact that because you have *learned* to think negatively, you can *unlearn* that negative thinking. Then you can *learn* new habits. Our job now is to help you learn to identify when you are thinking negative thoughts, and change them into positive thoughts or good self-talk. This will result in a change in your behavior pattern.

To help you identify any personal beliefs that are negative, read over the following list of negative thoughts. Do *you* ever say these self-defeating things to yourself?

Rationalization of Behavior

1. Some things I do are terrible; and I should be punished for doing them.

2. It is easier for me to avoid something that is difficult for me. If I ignore it, it will go away.

3. I must be perfect, and if I don't achieve 100% of what I set out to do, I am a failure.

4. I must control everything; I cannot enjoy life without being in control at all times.

5. I am not responsible for my reactions, because I have no control over my emotions and feelings.

6. I am not responsible if my surroundings cause me to feel unhappy.

7. I always react negatively in a certain stressful situation, and I can never change.

8. I must be loved by everyone all the time.

9. Someone else needs to correct my compulsive, behavior because I can't change.

10. I feel sorry for myself when things don't go my way.

11. Other people make me unhappy. It's just terrible when things don't go my way.

12. When something upsets me, it's not fair to expect me to act rationally.

These negative, limiting thoughts or self-talk are combined with four basic needs that we all have:

- The need for approval or acceptance
- The need for certainty and security

- The need for comfort
- The need to succeed

You may want to lose all of your excess weight *right now* and immediately be successful, which *is* an unrealistic goal. No matter how positively you program yourself to think, losing weight is not an easy process. If it were easy, you would have done it long ago, right? But losing weight follows a positive thought process that can be learned with practice and time. You can change the way you think to counter negative self-thoughts. This is called "cognitive restructuring".

Countering Negative Self-talk

First, you need to identify whether or not you have negative thoughts. Second, you need to ask yourself if these thoughts are logical and sensible? For example, in your need to succeed, you may be thinking like the fourth behavior rationalization listed above, "I must be able to control everything perfectly." Now, really, just how logical is that? Do you actually know anyone who is perfectly in control of everything all the time? Is it sensible to think that any human being ever is? Third, you can reinterpret your thought and substitute a more attainable positive thought. For example, "I cannot control everything all the time, but I *can* control how I *react* in a given situation."

To summarize how you can counter negative self-talk, let me give you an example of how it can be done. Let's say you started your eating plan and exercised regularly.

You step on the scale after two weeks, and your weight has not gone down. Right away, you think a negative thought: "This is *just* not working, because I am not losing weight!" Instead, ask yourself if your clothes are fitting differently. Other people may have commented to you that you look good. Remind yourself of these observations and reflect that changing your body fat composition requires not focusing on the scale numbers.

Weight loss or no scale change can be a very emotional thing to some people. Nutrition counseling provides an objective, non-emotional perspective with reinforcement and encouragement for whatever awareness and change has occurred. The goal is to gradually learn to "let go" of old, negative thought patterns and substitute positive behaviors.

Another strategy, which may be helpful in countering negative self-talk, is the "Behavior Chain." This can be diagrammed as shown on the following page. Picture your eating behavior as a *chain of events.* The first step is to identify the various links in the chain. Since we want to break the chain and change your behavior, we look for the weakest link. This would be the behavior area that appears to be the easiest to change first.

For our example, we will use the compulsive eating of cookies. Let us suppose that you went out shopping, and you bought a package of your favorite cookies "in case I have company." You leave the cookies sitting on the kitchen counter. It is the weekend and you are home alone with nothing to do on Saturday night; everyone else has something to do, and you don't (poor you), and so on. You are tired and bored. Feeling an urge to eat, you wander out to the kitchen. You see the package of cookies and take them back with you to where you are watching television.

Just one or two cookies, what could it hurt? Shouldn't you entitled to a little pleasure on Saturday night? So you eat two cookies while watching a sitcom, then, without thinking about it, you polish of the rest of them. When you look down and see the empty package, you start to feel guilty, and then you feel a sense of failure for opening the cookies in the first place. In this negative state, you feel that since you've already "blown it", you might as well "blow it" some more. So you go back to the kitchen to find something else to eat.

BEHAVIOR CHAIN

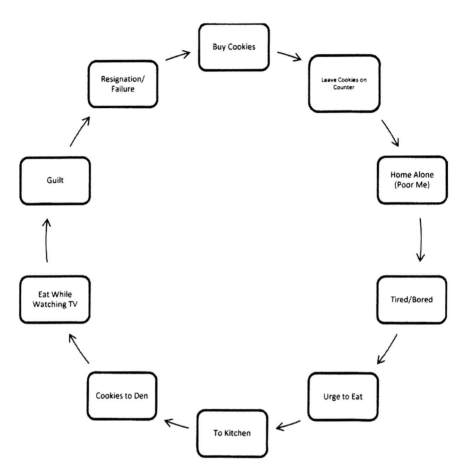

Your chain may look somewhat different than this, but the idea is the same. The weakest link in the above chain may be buying the cookies in the first place. For someone else, the weak link might be staying at home. Breaking the chain will alter the events that follow, link by link. Following is a new chain with positive changes in behavior.

POSITIVE BEHAVIOR CHAIN

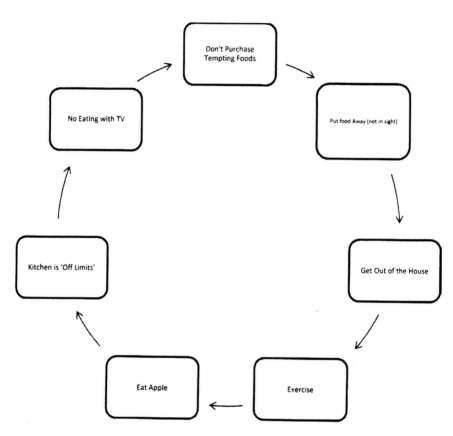

Your main task now is to practice substituting positive thoughts for the old negative ones and breaking the chain of events that have led to old behavior patterns. The more you practice, the easier it will become. You will need to practice these new thoughts and patterns of behavior for at least six months before they will become automatic. It takes persistent and consistent practice in order to estab-lish a new habit pattern that is conducive to achieving and *keeping* your new slim image.

Chapter 14

How Can You Be in Control of Your Life?

Being assertive allows you to maintain control over your behavior. Assertiveness is being able to openly express your true feelings in a positive manner, within the context of other people's feelings and rights. This in turn leaves you feeling better about yourself and more apt to be successful in resolving problems, including controlling your weight. It's important to realize that being assertive is not the same as being aggressive. Being assertive allows you to build confidence and success.

Being aggressive allows you to try and exert control over someone else's behavior. Aggression almost always leads to adverse and bitter reactions. The aggressive person may ignore the rights of others and is offensive. Other characteristics of someone who is being aggressive may include being: dishonest, hostile, defensive, insecure, sarcastic, rigid, abusive, uncaring, pushy, or frustrated.

The qualities of an assertive person may include being: honest, confident, flexible, caring, feeling good about oneself, capable, relaxed, sincere, and successful. These are the qualities you want to work to develop in yourself.

Perhaps you're not surrounded so much by aggressive people as you are by manipulative people. A manipulator is someone who attempts to use you or undermine you in order to get his or her way or to be in control. The manipulator may say, "You'll gain it all back, just like before." Or, "You've been so good, you deserve a treat." Or, "Can't you just have just a small piece of cake? You know I made it just for you."

Why do people do these things? In general, most people do not like change in their own lives or, surprisingly, in your life either. This is because their self-constructed and self-subsidized "security" (food, alcohol, relationships, nicotine, etc.) is threatened when you no longer seem to be subsidizing your security with food. They may also be jealous, or afraid they will have to compete with others for your affection. They may even fear that they will have to compete with you for others' attention!

In bribing you with your favorite foods, they may be looking for your weaknesses to regain control over your life. When you are not assertive, you become the victim of the manipulator. You allow *them* to make choices for *you*. The following "Bill of Rights" from Peter G. Lindner, M.D. will help you resist the manipulator. Once you learn that you have these rights, you must then assert yourself.

1. You have the right to set your *own* priorities so you can take control of your life.

2. You have the right to say "no" without feeling guilty.

3. You have the right to be taken seriously and listened to.

4. You have the right to your own opinion and to express your feelings.

5. You have the right to be treated with respect by others.

6. You have the right to make a mistake.

7. You have the right to ask for information and explanations.

8. You have the right to receive what you want when you pay for it.

9. You have the right to ask for what you want, even when you don't pay for it (at a party for example), realizing you may be refused.

10. You have the right *not* to assert yourself at all times.

Feeling better about yourself is a crucial ingredient of successful weight control.

To *feel* different, you need to *act* different..

One technique for practicing assertive skills regarding your desire to eat right and eat well is called the "parrot technique." You simply state what you want to say to express your feelings and then repeat it over and over again. Remember to speak in a calm voice. You do not need to expand on or explain your statement, and you ignore all statements made by the manipulator. If she/he was not ignoring your statements, you would not have to keep repeating them. She/he will run out of things to say in her/his attempt to manipulate you. If you persist in repeating your statement, she/he will abandon her/his attempts.

For example, when refusing a certain food, simply say, "No thank you, I don't care for any," over and over again. You do *not* need to explain why you *don't want any,* nor do you need to say, "Well, maybe I will try just a little taste," just to be polite. Simply smile calmly and repeat the same statement over and over.

Another technique is to appear to agree with the manipulator. The strategy here is to listen to the exact words the manipulator is using. You respond to what is actually being said, not to what you think the statement implies. This means you will agree with only one of the following:

1. Truth—if the statement is true.

2. Principle—if in principle the statement is accurate.

3. Possibility—if it is possible that what he is saying is accurate.

Do *not* try to justify your behavior or be aggressive. Used successfully, this strategy should eliminate any further negative remarks.

For example, if someone says, "You ate the dessert again, and you know that's not on your diet." You could respond with "truth," where you could say, "Why, yes, that's true. I did eat the dessert again." You could respond "in principle," by saying "You are right, I did. But I expect to eat desserts occasionally." You could respond as "possibility" by saying "You are probably right, I would lose better if I didn't eat it."

Both of these methods, the "parrot" method or the "agreement" method, will stop manipulators, but you must work to practice them regularly. As you practice these strategies with specific situations, you will become more assertive, and it will become easier for you to do. As you learn to believe that you can express your feelings in an assertive manner, your self-respect will increase. You will finally be in *control* of your own behavior.

As you can see, there are several reasons why your interpersonal relationships may change as you learn how to lose weight successfully. These relationships may actually improve over time and be more satisfying because you will be doing what you really want to do, but were afraid to do and say before.

Chapter 15

How to Understand Food Labels

Reading food labels can be an overwhelming task. However, there is a method of evaluating the contents, which should make it easier for you to incorporate some convenience or combination foods into your daily meal plan.

Analyzing a food label requires a two-fold approach. First, look at the picture of the product and estimate the portion sizes you believe are illustrated. Next, read the list of ingredients, which will be listed in descending order of concentration within the product. The item present in the largest amount will be listed first, then the next most available item, and so on.

As you review this list of ingredients, you will need to remember the macro nutrient distribution from the food groups represented in the Food Guide (Chapter 5). They are presented below to help you in your analysis.

Macronutrients in Food Groups

Food Group	CHO (g)	PRO (g)	Fat (g)
Nonfat milk	12	8	
Low fat protein		7	4
Bread/cereal	15	3	
Fruit	15		
Vegetable	5	2	
Fat			5

Your goal is to determine the "best fit" of food groups for a particular product. Use the picture of the product if it is available, and then look at the list of ingredients. Select the food group where the first listed ingredient would likely be found. For example, if the label lists the ingredients in this order: mushrooms, rice, whey protein, select the vegetable group as the first "best fit." Then estimate the number of servings present. It is helpful to write this down in a "matrix form" as presented below. Then go to the food group represented by the second ingredient on the list (in our example, rice) and estimate the number of servings present and so on.

Continue to do this until you have satisfied the major foods represented. You will end up with a listing similar to that below:

	Food Group	CHO (g)	PRO (g)	FAT (g)
mushrooms	1 vegetable	5	2	
rice	1 bread/cereal	15	3	
whey protein	½ milk	6	4	
Totals:		26	9	

Compare your list of numbers to that on the label. Your goal is to have the numbers in close agreement with the label. (You may have to revise your estimates to accomplish this.) You will then have an idea of how to incorporate this item into your meal plan. The above example is similar to products sold as substitutes for hamburger patties. The picture in this case might lead you to believe that the product would be a major protein source. However, our analysis suggests that it would supply only a small amount of quality protein. That is, you cannot quickly look at the protein grams on a label, divide by 7 (1 oz. quality protein = 7 grams protein) and come up with ounces of quality protein. In our example, over half the protein grams come from lower quality or incomplete sources (5 grams from vegetable and grain).

If the food label provides you with more detailed information, for example "Exchanges," you will not need to do this exercise. The word "exchange" on a food label means "choice," and is used to identify the same food categories that were described earlier in the Food Guide. The manufacturer has provided the label information based on an analysis of how the item is formulated. However, this exercise can be good practice for you. You can compare your results with those listed as the "exchanges." There may be some discrepancies, but that does not mean you are doing it wrong. Because the food manufacturer knows the exact formula in producing the product. For example, the amount of starch used to thicken a sauce will affect the carbohydrate grams; we have no way of estimating that contribution so there may be some differences.

Now, let us work together through an example, using "Healthy Choice™ Chicken a l'Orange." The label describes it as "tender chicken breast meat with orange sauce and rice with carrots," 260 calories and a weight of 9 oz. The picture of this particular product shows a chicken breast in three slices (about 3 oz.) on about 1/2 cup rice with a few flakes of carrot for color.

The ingredient list is as follows:

"Chicken Pouch: cooked chicken breast meat, water, modified food starch, flavoring, salt, water, orange juice concentrate, brown sugar, modified food starch, chicken fat, flavorings, spices, maltodextrin. Rice pouch: cooked white rice, carrots, cooked wild rice, soybean oil."

The nutritional information per serving is:

Serving size   9 oz.

Calories   260

Carbohydrate (g) 39

Protein (g) 22

Fat (g) 2

The information on polyunsaturated fat, saturated fat, cholesterol, fiber, sodium, and potassium is omitted since we will not be using it in our analysis. However, if sodium is a concern to you, you may want to look for those products with a lower value on sodium.

> **¼ tsp. of salt = 500 mg. sodium**
> **To estimate how much salt/sodium is added in processing divide the mg. by 500**

To estimate the best fit, let's start with the protein group since chicken is the first ingredient. How many ounces will provide us with about 22 grams? Remember that rice is also an ingredient and 3 g of protein are provided per serving of grain. Thus, we will want to allow for some protein to come from bread and/or vegetable food groups.

Analysis of Healthy Choice™ Chicken a l' Orange

Food Item	CHO (g)	PRO (g)	FAT (g)
2 oz. chicken (2 PRO)		14	6
1/2 cup rice (1 CHO)	15	3	
1/4 cup carrot (1/2 VEG)	2.5	1	
TOTALS:	17.5	18	6
LABEL READS:	39	22	2

At this point, we have more than satisfied the fat content; the extra 4 grams (our total of 6 grams minus 2 grams fat on label = 4 grams) are not significant. Thus, we have over-estimated the fat contribution. Remember we used a general value of 3 grams fat per ounce of chicken. In this case the fat content of the chicken breast is less. Thus, this product is very low in fat and certainly does not have any added fat.

We are low in carbohydrate grams at 17.5 vs. 39, but we are close in protein at 18 vs. 22. Now, we must decide how to make up the difference. At this point it may be helpful to go back to the food label ingredient list. Since modified food starch is listed a couple of times, we need to allow for this contribution to the carbohydrate figures on the label. Orange juice concentrate and brown sugar are also listed, which are additional sources of carbohydrate. However, since they are not present at a significant amount, we cannot justify allowing for a fruit serving. Therefore, let's see how many more bread or starch servings it takes to match our numbers to the label. Adding 1-1/2 bread servings give us the closest estimate of exchanges or food choices:

Food Item	CHO (g)	PRO (g)	FAT (g)
Values from above	17.5	18	6
add			
1--1/2 bread (1-1/2 CHO)	22.5	4.5	
OUR TOTALS:	40	22.5	6
Vs.			
PRODUCT LABEL:	39	22	2

In summary then, we have determined that this product would contain 2 oz. meat (2 PRO), 2-1/2 servings bread (2-1/2 CHO), and 1/2 serving vegetable (1/2 VEG). The label states it provides 1-1/2 oz. lean meat, 2 bread, and 1-1/2 vegetable servings. You can see that we over-estimated protein slightly and the visual estimation was way off (3 oz. vs. 1-1/2 oz.). The discrepancy in vege-tables (1/2 serving vs. 1-1/2 servings) may result from how the manufacturer values and quantifies the food starch, etc.

We have derived the "best fit" in our estimation. When using this product, I would recommend that you add another serving of vegetable and or salad to complete the menu, since the amount of carrot is limited.

When you practice this exercise over and over, it will seem much simpler. You can also use this strategy for analyzing meals served in group settings (potlucks, restau-rants, etc.). You are estimating as close as possible how the foods served break down in macronutrients (CHO—carbohydrate, PRO—protein, FAT—fat).

Based on that information, you are also able to determine the "best fit" in food groups to your plan.

Chapter 16
Menu Planning

Planning menus is one of the most helpful tools to eating well. Studies have shown that most people don't decide what to have for dinner until after four in the afternoon. It is no wonder that today's grocery stores have turned into "take-out restaurants." All this comes at a greater cost—financially and calorically. Think about the meals you may be in the habit of picking up on your way home— pizza, Chinese or Thai take-out, prepared ready-to-heat items, pre-cooked ribs, chicken, or turkey. Some of these items may be acceptable on an occasional basis, but the fat and sodium content can be significant. In addition, the amount and variety of brightly colored vegetables and whole grain choices is lacking.

EASY STEPS FOR MENU PLANNING

Take about thirty minutes once a week for this task. Once you have experience you may find that ten to fifteen minutes is all you need. You may also want to use the weekly grocery ads to plan meals around specials of the week in meats and produce. Many families use about ten recipes or variations thereof, so the process does not need to be complicated.

Start with two sheets of paper large enough to include your shopping list and the days of the week---8 1/2" by 11" is a good size. One sheet needs to have the meals you are planning for across the top and the days of the week down the side. On each day you might indicate any additional demands on your time that will affect the time you have for meal preparation, for example, children's after school activities, evening meetings, work hours, etc.

The recipes in the appendix provide you with some additional ideas for putting your menu plan into practice. Feel free to use any recipe you like. You now know how to evaluate it using the skills we reviewed in Chapter 15. The Food Guide information in the Appendix may also be helpful to use at this time. It illustrates a variety of foods in each category. Seeing the many foods to choose from may help you in creative menu planning.

Menu Planning Worksheet

	Breakfast	Lunch	Dinner	Snacks
Monday				
Tuesday				
Wednesday				
Thursday				
Friday				
Saturday				
Sunday				

The aisles of the grocery store can be used to organize your shopping list. This allows you to move more efficiently through the store. For example, start in the first aisle to your left on entering the store. This may be where you find fresh fruits and vegetables. When you are first organizing your shopping list, you may want to outline the order of the aisles. The outline can then be duplicated for future use. Just hope your store does not move things around too frequently! My favorite store totally remodeled over a six-month period of time. Every week foods would be moved from one location to another. The employees were as frustrated as the shoppers were during the ordeal. Now that it is complete and somewhat stable, it's easier to find things. Once that your outline is ready, follow these easy steps for menu planning.

Shopping List

Fruit/Vegetables	Bread
Spices/Baking Mixes	Canned Fruit/Veg.
Butter/Dairy/Egg	Fresh Meat/Poultry
Salad Dressing/Pickles	Cereal
Magazines/Household	Bakery/Deli
Pet Supplies	Frozen Foods

START WITH PROTEIN-RICH FOODS

Start with the protein-rich foods for each day. For example, Monday breakfast might be lean ham, lunch might be tuna, and dinner will be planned with beef. After you jot down the types of protein you want to plan around, you then go back and decide how you want to prepare it. This will help you keep the choices varied and you can "plan ahead" to have some foods cooked ahead to save time on a hectic day. You may also include portion sizes to help you follow your meal pattern. This step also helps you with the amounts you need to purchase. For example, if you are feeding four individuals, you would buy 1 lb. lean beef to yield four 3-oz. portions.

At breakfast, the ham may be planned with toast. The next time ham is included on a menu, you may use it with eggs as a frittata. The tuna may be served with a fresh tomato in summer or made into a grilled sandwich on a cold day. The beef could vary from a roast on a Sunday, when there is time to prepare it, to fajitas when you need something in a hurry. As you develop your menu, be sure to jot down on your shopping list what you need to buy. Some ingredients you will have on hand. Before shopping, it's always a good idea to check the supplies of staples (flour, sugar, herbs and spices, etc.) to eliminate extra trips to the store. This saves both time and money.

ADDING FRUITS and VEGETABLES

Step two includes adding fruits and vegetables. You may want to refer to the Food Guide in the Appendix to assist you with variety. You should include both vitamin A and C sources daily. Foods rich in these nutrients are indicated for you to choose readily.

The actual form they will take will come as the menu develops. For example, you might prepare oven roasted beef, carrots, onion and potato, while the next time the beef is fajitas with red, yellow, and orange peppers added as the vegetables of choice. Remember four servings or more of vegetables each day is optimal.

INCLUDING DAIRY PRODUCTS

The next category to include is dairy products. If your meal plan eliminates these for any reason, you will need to include more quality protein and calcium sources. You may vary the source from milk used with cereal to milk used as an ingredient in a recipe.

ADDING GRAINS and CEREALS

The last category of foods to add is cereals and grains. These are generally the simplest for everyone to include. A slice of whole wheat bread goes with our ham at breakfast, followed with whole grain crackers accompanying our tuna salad. Dinner already includes a potato, so we may decide to add 'light' popcorn as an evening snack.

COLOR, TEXTURE, and VARIETY

Once you have completed filling in the food categories for each day, it is a good idea to review the overall menu plan. First, check for color. A nutritious menu where everything is white is not very appetizing. For example, visualize poached chicken breast, mashed potato, and cauliflower. Would that appeal to you? Baking the chicken with a crumb coating would add color. Substituting a baked sweet potato for the mashed potato would add additional contrast. With these changes, the cauliflower would be acceptable, or we could substitute broccoli for the cauliflower for even more color.

Next, think about texture. Suppose you had a tuna sandwich on soft white bread with canned pears. How appetizing does that menu sound? Think about how a combination of soft and crunchy foods adds interest to a meal. Using whole grain bread adds color and texture as well as nutrients. A fresh red pear or apple adds color and texture.

Overall variety in your menu is important. The more varied our food choices, the more likely we are to obtain the fifty-plus nutrients we need every day. Some individuals need more variety than others. For example, if I encourage someone to add quality protein, such as lean ham, at breakfast, they may respond a couple of weeks later that they are bored with their choices. When asked what they would rather have, they may respond with cereal. They can have cereal every day and not be bored!

Your menu plan should remain flexible. For example, even though you planned a specific menu for any given day doesn't mean you cannot change it. Let's say an activity comes up on the Sunday you planned the beef roast and there was no time to cook it. You could switch to Monday's dinner menu, and put the roast in a slow cooker for Monday evening.

The principle goal behind the menu plan is to have all the groceries you need in the house for any given week. Plan. Buy. Prepare. Enjoy!

BON APPÉTIT!

Chapter 17

What do you do when eating out?

Eating out in restaurants presents a particular challenge when you are trying to change old habits. The answer is not to deprive yourself of the enjoyment of a nice lunch or dinner in a restaurant; rather, the answer is to plan ahead. When you know you are going out to dinner, you may want to eat lighter during the day. Do *not* make the mistake of not eating all day and then going out to dinner or a party "starving" hungry. This is asking for a problem, as it is very difficult to eat with restraint when everything looks and smells irresistible! Try eating some low fat protein with vegetables and a non-caloric drink earlier in the day, and save your bread and fruit choices for eating out.

Today, many restaurants and fast food establishments offer "lighter fare" menu options with nutrition information available. It is possible that the food served may have more calories and fat than indicated, but it is generally 'lighter' than the regular fare. More and more, it is possible to eat fast food wisely. You can ask how foods are prepared, portioned, etc. Ordering food in a restaurant is one place you can practice your assertive skills. For example, you can ask that sauces be left off or served to the side, or that the meat be broiled rather than fried.

Another very simple hint is to always ask for salad dressing on the side. You then can add as little as possible to satisfy your taste. An even more effective method is to dip your fork into the dressing and then into the greens. You will find that you require very little dressing this way and the calorie and fat savings are significant.

Since you are eating smaller portions, another strategy is to order a la carte or smaller portions when they are available. You might order an appetizer and a salad in lieu of a complete dinner. Depending on the restaurant, this may be just the right amount.

If you are very disciplined, you can customize your portion of food after it is served and before you start to eat. You know from experience how the proportions look when you eat at home according to your menu pattern, so portion off those same amounts in the restaurant; take the remaining food home for another meal. Asking for a take-out box at the time you are served will make this easier. This makes dining out more economical—two or more meals for the price of one, and you don't have to cook!

Another, similar method, is to eat one half of everything, and then take the remaining half home. This also takes discipline and practice. If your discipline is not strong enough to do this, you might try making half of the portions on your plate inedible by pouring lots of salt and/or pepper on it. Then if your resolve weakens as you are eating, you will be stopped short by the unacceptable taste.

Set a reasonable goal for yourself. When you are first practicing eating out, try it once a week. As you gain confidence in your ability to make wise choices, you may go out more often. During the holidays, most of us have many social functions to attend which seem to involve high calorie food. During those times, a reasonable goal may be to maintain your weight rather than lose weight. The typical person gains three to seven pounds during this time, so if you maintain your weight you are doing great!

Again, I caution you to be realistic about your goals. When attending a cocktail party, your plan may be to limit your beverage to a non-alcoholic, non-caloric choice. When you are holding a glass in your hand, even the most solicitous host or hostess will be satisfied. You do not have to tell anyone what you are drinking. If you think that the snacks may be particularly tempting, have a protein-containing snack before heading out. It also helps to position yourself away from the food tables. Do not expect perfection. Know that you have not failed if you eat a few nuts or some chips with dip. However, do know that there is a *big* difference when you eat a whole can of nuts or a whole bowl of dip!

Look at every dining out experience as an opportunity to practice your new skills. Make a plan and write it down in advance of the occasion, and then use your visualization skills to rehearse your plan. Think about some of your assertive options, such as asking if you can order first when the server comes to take orders. This is one way to not be influenced by the choices of others.

If you have a particularly hard time with the warm basket of bread or chips, either remove them from the table or at least from your side of the table. If you choose to spend one of your bread servings on tortilla chips, take a handful out of the basket and place them on a plate or napkin. Then place the basket out of your reach. Remember that salsa is a very acceptable low calorie dip, as opposed to onion dip or guacamole.

These hints apply whether you are eating out at a restaurant or as a guest in someone's home. You can always call the hostess ahead of time to ask what she is serving. Then you can choose whether to explain (being assertive is very liberating!) that you would like to plan your other food for the day to make sure you can include all of the wonderful cooking in your daily eating plan. Then make your plans accordingly.

Be very low-key about whatever you choose to ask or tell your hostess. There is nothing worse than making an "issue" of your "diet." This can set you up for someone to sabotage you, either by monitoring what you put in your mouth or by pushing food on you that you don't want. Many times, it is just better to be quiet and make the best choices you can. You can discuss at a later time with your Registered Dietitian or counselor how you handled the situation. You may learn another strategy, which you can practice the next time you are eating out.

PRACTICAL HINTS

Fast Food

Look for salads or broiled lean meat/poultry sandwiches (be aware of special sauces, dressing, or mayonnaise if necessary). Deep-fried fish sandwiches are very high in fat. Side salads with low calorie dressings add servings of vegetables and satisfy the need for "crunch" in place of chips or fries. Be sure to use a small amount of dressing; one half a package or less should be plenty. Try the method of dipping the fork into the dressing before picking up the greens.

Mexican

Look for fajitas—beef, chicken, or shrimp cooked with tomato, onion, and bell pepper, and ask that they not be cooked in oil. Try to always choose items that include vegetables. Go light on sour cream and guacamole. Remember to budget your carbohydrate (CHO) choices—chips, refried beans, rice, and tortillas can add up quickly.

Chinese

Most dishes will include small amounts of meat, fish, or poultry combined with a variety of vegetables. Look for dishes prepared with very little oil. Steamed rice will be lightest in fat. Fried rice and chow mein noodles add to fat and carbohydrate. Sweet and sour dishes are generally high in sugar and fat.

Italian

Look for entrées with tomato sauce, as opposed to Alfredo (white) sauce. Dishes drenched with the latter are high in fat and low in quality protein. Chicken, veal, or fish dishes prepared with vegetables (tomato, mushroom, etc.) are good choices. If you want pasta, remember to factor it into your protein and carbohydrate quota for the day. Since the garlic bread may be too hard for you to pass up, save up some of your fat and carbohydrate for the day so you can enjoy a piece (practice having a *piece*, not the whole basket!) with your meal.

French

Look for entrées with a "novelle" preparation method. In this case, the base for the sauce is generally a pureed vegetable rather than the high fat butter/cream/cheese sauce found in so many French dishes. Many quality French restaurants also serve modest portions.

Bon Appetit!

Enjoy yourself when eating out. Think about how much fun it is to be in control while eating out! When you concentrate on your company and ambiance, your meal should be a leisurely and positive experience. Once again, with best wishes, bon appétit!

Chapter 18

Keys to Continued Success

Maintenance is the most important stage of the weight loss process. Once you have attained your goal of body fat composition and weight, you are ready to appreciate the fine art of balancing your food skills for the rest of your life, while you remain in control, assertive and happy.

E = eating

A = attitude

T = training/exercise

These three components must always stay in "balance" to help you maintain your lower weight. This aspect of the E.A.T. process continues, but not to worry! You have been training and preparing yourself to recognize that this is one of the best things you have ever decided to do for yourself.

You are not on a "diet" that limits your choices. You have learned how to choose foods to eat that are right for *you*. You have learned how to eat discretionary calories and stay in control. You have learned how important exercise is to your program. You have learned what your "eating problems" are and successful ways to solve them.

Dangerous Curves Ahead

Let's hope that all curves ahead are sitting prettily or handsomely on your body. If not, you can handle them by preparing yourself now. There are a variety of circumstances, that have been identified with relapsing or regaining lost weight.

- Depression or a major life change (death of a spouse, divorce, loss of a job, illness)
- Socializing (frequent traveling or entertaining; eating meals away from home)
- Testing or pushing the "outer" limits (exposing oneself to tempting food, having no structured eating pattern, vacations, holidays, etc.)

Be on the lookout for these, so that at the first sign of difficulty, you take some positive action while you are still in control.

Smooth Sailing

The factors, which help most with successful maintenance, are a positive sense of well-being and emotional satisfaction. Personal motivation is also high on the list, as is a commitment to follow through and accomplish what you have set out to do. The positive changes in your body will be very helpful in maintaining motivation. Not to mention new ease in buying and wearing clothing, a more youthful appearance, and improved risk factors for good health.

Any support you receive from family and friends will, of course, be very encouraging to you. However, understand that after you maintain your goal weight for a period of time, people will stop making comments. You need to learn to depend on your own inner strength, personal satisfaction, and determination to motivate you to continue maintaining your weight. With all the attention you may have experienced as your weight was coming off, you may have learned to encourage yourself with others' words. It may not seem so easy to continue working at your goal when no one seems to notice anymore. Therefore, encourage yourself mentally and through self-talk, to be self-sustaining and independent of any need for others' comments and encouragement. You can still enjoy and relish encouragement and compliments when they come, but you will not *need* them to continue to succeed. Be ever resolved that you are doing and have done it all for *you*, and you alone.

There are two additional tools to help you sustain your efforts: reassessing your body composition by being alert to how your clothes fit and keeping a maintenance graph.

Maintaining Body Fat Composition

First, your goal is to maintain your ideal body fat composition. Your clothes provide the simplest feedback for you. Be alert to the way your jeans, slacks, or dresses fit. They should fit as comfortably as when you first reached your goal.

Another strategy for maintaining your ideal body fat is to have it re-measured periodically. For the first year, I suggest re-measuring every three months. Thereafter, it may be helpful for you to continue being measured on occasion to reinforce your accomplishment. For some that will mean continuing quarterly. For others, it may mean one or two times a year.

Maintenance Graph

The Maintenance Graph is similar to the exercise graph you have used up to now. However, since you are working to maintain your weight, the bottom part of the graph is divided into three weight ranges and works like a traffic light system:

"Green" or Safe Range = the bottom 3 lbs. is defined as your ideal body weight range

"Yellow" or Caution Range = the next 3 lbs. up on the graph

"Red" or Stop Range = the remaining pounds above the Caution zone

The Maintenance Graph is based on the same principles we used earlier. Your protein intake is fixed and your fat intake remains low at a maximum of 30% calories from fat. The variable you will adjust is the CHO (carbohydrate) servings.

As you transition to maintenance, you will be advised to increase 1/2 CHO serving (7-8 grams carbohydrate) per day for four or five days. If your weight is stable, you will increase another 1/2 serving (7-8 grams) for an additional four or five days. You will continue to increase CHO servings as long as your weight stabilizes and stays within the Green Zone. This gradual process allows your body to rehydrate slowly as you adjust for increased carbohydrate servings.

Remember that carbohydrates end up as water and carbon dioxide after all is said and done.

As you weigh yourself, your goal in maintenance is to stay in the "Green" or safe zone. If an occasion arises that leads you to make undesirable choices and you increase your CHOs quickly, you will note an immediate increase on the scale. Remember this is related to fluid rather than fat balance. It can take as many as seven days for your weight to go back to the previous level. Remind yourself that you *know* there is no reason to panic because of what you have learned.

Using this graph allows you to make adjustments to stay in control. Continue to graph your exercise as you did earlier.

This tool provides tremendous visual reinforce-ment and may be something you want to continue long-term.

MAINTENANCE GRAPH

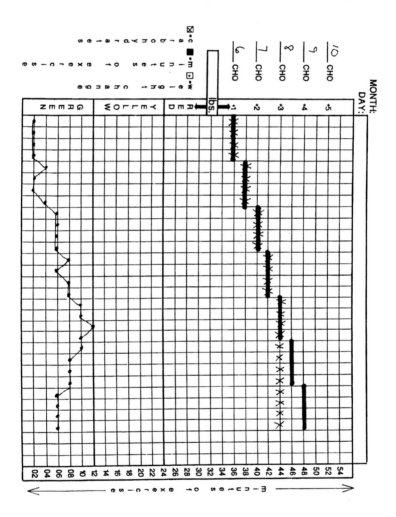

Ten Key Points to Continued Success

In conclusion, there are ten key points that will contribute to your success:

1. You expect to be successful.

2. You are self-motivated.

3. You have a positive self-image and always try to look your best.

4. You are self-directed and set daily and long-term goals.

5. You are in control and actively work to make positive change.

6. You are disciplined, as you regularly practice your new habit patterns.

7. You see yourself thinner and are determined to stay that way.

8. You take one day at a time.

9. You recognize your potential and strive to be the best you can be.

10. You communicate your ideas and feelings with others; you are assertive without being manipulative.

Remember that you are unique, and you *can* lose weight and achieve an appropriate body composition with the correct combination of foods and activity. There are multiple reasons why people become overweight, but most weight-reduction programs just address the food calories a person consumes. Your E.A.T. program considers all the important aspects of your lifestyle that affect your body weight. As you realize by now, it is not just the food one eats.

It is lifestyle and behavior in balance that brings success. When your lifestyle and behaviors are changed, the weight loss stays changed as well.

Your weight issue is not the same as everyone else's—some do eat a lot while others do not. In addition to the composition of food that you eat, the nutritive composition must be optimal based on the standards known at the time. Nutrition is a young science; however, we will continue to learn more. Always maintain an interest in staying abreast of these changes and how they may apply to you. Remember to keep exercising as well.

Your goal is to keep your eating, attitude, training or exercise (E.A.T. model) in balance forever. Learning to be healthy is an ongoing "process", a positive, effective, doable process that benefits every area of your life. It is a lifelong investment you are making in your health and well-being, as well as, your physical appearance. This is the "secret" to maintenance.

Appendix

THE FOOD GUIDE

Protein (PRO)

The foods on this list supply an average of 6 to 7 grams of protein and low, medium and high amounts of fat. The overall goal should be to average 3 grams of fat per ounce of protein consumed. Use the chart below to choose most of your protein sources from those that are low in fat. Some choices could be medium fat, but few should be high in fat. For example, if you want to have sausage for breakfast—which is high in fat at 11 grams per ounce of cooked sausage, you should choose lower fat sources of protein through the rest of the day. For example, you might have two ounces of white water-packed tuna and 1/2 cup lowfat cottage cheese, which would give you a total of 12.5 grams of fat or an average of 2.5 grams fat per the five ounces total protein for the day. These foods are generally good sources of vitamin B-6, iron, and zinc.

Table: One ounce cooked portion of protein foods

LOW FAT: 25 calories, 0 fat	40 calories, 1.5 g fat
abalone	cod
clams	haddock
crab, shrimp	Canadian bacon
shrimp	tuna, white in water
¼ cup low fat	3 Tbsp. Nutlettes
¼ cup cottage cheese	
1/3 cup Greek yogurt	

MEDIUM: FAT 50-60 calories, 2 g fat	70-80 calories, 5.5 g fat
sole, flounder	lean pork
veal	mozzarella, part skim
halibut	¼ cup part skim ricotta
salmon	1 large egg
sardine in brine	3.5 oz tofu
lean beef (flank steak)	liver
ground sirloin	¼ cup edamame
lean lamb	3 Tbsp soynuts
poultry, no skin	1 Tbsp hemp seed

HIGH FAT: 90-100 calories, 9 g fat	130 calories, 11 g fat
ground chuck	pork sausage
cheddar cheese	pepperoni
jack cheese	paté
American cheese	3 Tbsp. nuts/seeds

Remember that when you select luncheon meats and cheese you should look for low fat products, which means the grams of fat per ounce should be 5 grams or less. For example, the label on a poultry bologna may say "96% fat free" and each slice, which weighs 2/3 ounce, provides 4 grams of protein and 4 grams of fat. On a "first look", you may feel this is a good choice. However, to substitute the poultry bologna for an ounce of lean protein, you would need to eat one and one-half slices to get the protein up to 6 grams; as a result, the fat content is now 6 grams. This type of product should be selected carefully by evaluating what the label really means. To compare it to our earlier example, five ounces of poultry bologna would supply 30 grams of fat for the day—more than twice the total when we planned on one ounce of sausage with other low fat protein sources (12.5 grams fat).

Starch (CHO)

This group of foods includes breads, cereals and grains. These foods supply starch (carbohydrate), protein, vitamins and minerals. Whole grain products are good sources of fiber; they also contain thiamin, niacin, folate, vitamin E, iron, phosphorus, magnesium, zinc, and other trace minerals. Some products may be enriched (meaning that thiamin, riboflavin, niacin, and iron are added back after processing), but they tend to be lower in fiber. Other products, such as ready-to-eat cereal, may be fortified with additional nutrients.

Table: One serving supplies an average of 80 calories with 15 g carbohydrate and 3 g protein. The (A) indicates good source of Vitamin A.

Starches and Starchy Vegetables

½ cup peas, corn, hominy

½ cup lentils, beans (omit 1 PRO)

½ cup white or sweet(A) potato

½ large ear corn

3 cups fat free popcorn

1/3 cup rice, pasta, couscous

1 cup winter squash(A)

2/3 cup lima beans

1 cup non-cream soup

½ cup bulgur

Breads and Crackers

¼ large bagel

½ English muffin, pita

4 breadsticks

½ hamburger/hotdog bun

¾ oz. matzo or pretzels

24 oyster crackers

8 animal crackers

2 rice cakes

1 small slice bread (80 cal)

2 slices light bread

10 wheat thins

5 low fat triscuits

6 soda or saltines

1 small flour or corn tortilla

3 graham cracker squares

Cereals

3 Tbsp. wheat bran

½ cup All Bran

¾ cup flake cereal

¼ cup grape nuts, low fat granola

½ cup cooked cereal

1-1/2 cups puffed cereal

Miscellaneous with Added Fat

2-1/2 inch biscuit

1/5 regular muffin

½ cup ice milk/ice cream

1 oz cookie

1 cup cream soup

¾ oz croutons

1 oz chocolate

¼ cup sorbet (fat free)

Fruit (CHO)

This group of foods supplies us with fiber when the fruit is consumed rather than juice. One serving per day should be a good source of Vitamin C. Fruits high in this vitamin are marked with a (C). Since the carbohydrate content (15 g) is the same as for starch, you may be allowed to interchange these servings. Some fruits are good sources of Vitamin A; note that they are indicated by an (A) following the fruit.

Table: One serving supplies an average of 60 calories and 15 g carbohydrate; the portion is ½ cup unless otherwise indicated.

1 cup Boysenberry, blackberry, strawberry(C), blueberry, raspberry, honeydew, cantaloupe (C)(A)	
apple	applesauce
apricot (A)	banana
cherries	fig
fruit cocktail (in juice)	grapefruit (C)
grapes	kiwi
orange (C)	papaya (C)(A)pear
peach	pear
persimmon (A)	pineapple
plum	
tangerine (C)	
dried fruit is concentrated since the water is gone, so the portion will weight ½ to 2/3 ounce.	

Vegetable (VEG)

The foods on this list are generally low in calories and you may eat them freely. You should definitely try to include a minimum of four servings daily, as almost all vegetables are important sources of fiber. Some vegetables are good sources of vitamin C and vitamin A; they are noted with (C) and (A) respectively. When eaten fresh or minimally cooked, the vitamin C and folate content will be preserved. Dark green vegetables are generally good sources of vitamin B-6, folate, and magnesium

Table: One serving supplies an average of 25 calories and 5 g carbohydrate and 2 g protein; one serving is ½ cup, cooked or raw. For raw leafy greens the portion is 1 cup

asparagus	artichoke
bamboo shoot	bell pepper (C)(A)
beet	bok choy (A)
broccoli (C)	Brussels sprouts (C)
cabbage (C)	carrot (A)
cauliflower (C)	celery
chard (A)	chili pepper (C)(A)
eggplant	greens (A)
green beans	green onion (A)
okra	onion
leaf lettuce (A)	head lettuce (iceburg)
mushrooms	spinach (A)
pumpkin (A)	summer squash
snow pea (C)	tomato (C)

Milk Products (CHO and PRO)

The foods included on this list provide at least 250 mg calcium, as well as supplying magnesium and zinc. They are also good sources of protein, riboflavin, thiamin, vitamin A, B-6, and B-12. Since fluid and dry milk are fortified, they are also good sources of vitamin D. Milk products may serve as the primary source of protein and vitamin B-12 for people consuming a vegetarian diet. If you are not a milk drinker, your meal pattern will have to be adjusted for its macro nutrient composition. You will also need to choose alternate calcium sources (see the table on page 49), or you may need to take a calcium supplement.

Table: One serving supplies 90 calories, 12 g carbohydrate and 8 g protein

3 Tbsp. nonfat dry milk solids
½ cup evaporated skim milk
1 cup skim or nonfat milk or buttermilk
1 cup plain nonfat yogurt

NOTE:

If you choose 1% milk, add 2.5 g fat and 23 calories

If you choose 2% milk, add 5 g fat and 45 calories

If you choose whole milk, add 10 g fat and 90 calories

If you cannot or do not drink milk, remember to add 1 oz. protein and 300 mg. calcium per cup.

Fat

The foods in the following list provide a concentrated source of calories. Remember that fat supplies 9 calories per gram. Fats supply fat-soluble vitamins A, D, and E, as well as the essential fatty acid, linoleic acid. Linoleic acid is called an essential fatty acid because it cannot be made in our body; we must obtain it in our food.

Fatty acids are the basic chemical units in fat. They are saturated, monounsaturated, or polyunsaturated depending on the amount of hydrogen they contain. (Remember our example earlier of the bus.) All dietary fats contain various amounts of these three types of fatty acids. Fats high in unsaturated fatty acids are good sources of vitamin E and linoleic acid. Thus, a minimum of three servings of fats high in polyunsaturated and monounsaturated fatty acids are recommended daily. In designing your meal pattern, you will want to limit the percentage of calories from fat in all foods to 30% or less of total calories.

Table: One serving supplies 45 calories and 5 g fat

Unsaturated Fats

1 tsp. margarine (first ingredient must be liquid oil
2 tsp. diet margarine (water is first ingredient
1 tsp. mayonnaise
10 medium green olives
6 medium ripe black olives
2 tsp. oil-based salad dressing
1/8 avocado
1 tsp canola, olive, safflower, corn, peanut, soybean, flax oil

Saturated Fats – minimize use of these

1 tsp. butter
¼ oz. salt pork
1 tsp. cream sauce, vegetable shortening
5 Tbsp. non-dairy whip topping
2 Tbsp shred coconut
1 Tbsp cream-based salad dressing
2 Tbsp. light cream, sour cream
1 Tbsp. whipping cream, cream cheese
1 slice bacon
½ oz chitterlings
1 tsp. coconut oil
2 Tbsp. coffee creamer
1 tsp. gravy, meat drippings, palm oil

Sugars and Discretionary Calories

Sugars supply mainly energy as calories with few additional nutrients. Many sweets also supply large amounts of fat. Since most of us who need and want to lose weight do not want to feel deprived, we may include some discretionary calories in your daily meal plan. These are divided into 150 calorie choices. Some examples include the following; additional choices may be added in consultation with your Registered Dietitian.

Discretionary Calories

1 oz. chocolate
1/16th (2 oz. pie)
½ oz. hard candy
2 oz. cake (approx. 1/24th)
6 oz. wine
1 oz. cookie (number depends on size)
6 oz. average mixed drink
1 oz. donut
1 granola bar (1 oz.)
12 oz. regular carbonated beverage
8 oz. wine cooler
12 oz. beer

Free Foods

The following foods may be consumed freely:

Sugar free gelatin
Clear broth or bouillon
Coffee
Tea
Club soda
Sugar free carbonated beverated
Pure spices and herbs
 Mineral water
2 Crystal Light or equal bars per day (14 calories each
and 2-3 g carbohydrate)

RECIPES

The recipes that follow are divided into categories for you to use as desired. The count indicated refers to the information in your personalized meal plan or that you may derive from the Food Guide (Appendix).

BEVERAGES

Frosty Cappuccino

1	cup 1% milk or soy milk
1	Tbsp. chocolate syrup
1	tsp. instant coffee powder
2	ice cubes

Blend all ingredients.

Yield: 2 servings   Count: 1 CHO 1/2 PRO

Frozen Mocha

1	cup nonfat chocolate milk or soy milk
1	Tbsp. instant espresso powder
2	tsp. cocoa powder
2	pkt. sugar substitute
1/4	tsp. vanilla extract
1	cup ice cubes

Add all ingredients to blender and process until smooth.

Yield: 2 servings   Count: 1/2 CHO 1/2 PRO

Herb Lemonade

1/2	cup Splenda
6	cups water
6	4 inch sprigs fresh rosemary or other herb (i.e. mint, basil, etc.)
1/2 - 3/4	cup fresh lemon juice

Bring 2 cups water and Splenda to boil. Add remaining ingredients and steep for 30 minutes. Strain out herb. Serve hot or cold.

Yield: 6 servings   Count: free

Hot Mocha

6	cups brewed coffee
1/2	cup sugar
1/2	cup unsweetened cocoa
6	Tbsp. Kahlua Coffee Liqueur (this alcohol addition may be omitted)

Combine coffee, sugar and cocoa in saucepan until hot (do not boil). Remove from heat and stir in Kahlua.

Yield: 10 servings   Count: 1 CHO

Mock Margarita

1-1/2	cups sparkling or mineral water
2	Tbsp. fresh lime juice
1-2	packets Splenda or sugar substitute of choice
1	egg white (dip egg in boiling water for 30 seconds before breaking)
1/2	cup crushed ice Ice cubes and lime slices for garnish

Pour water into blender. Add lime juice, sweetener, egg white and crushed ice. Blend until frothy. Rub lime around rims of chilled glasses. Fill each glass with ice cubes and the frothy margarita mixture. Garnish with lime.

Yield: 4 servings   Count: free

SOUPS

African Peanut Chicken Soup

4   boneless chicken breasts, cooked and diced
1   cup chopped onion
1   Tbsp. each minced garlic and curry powder
1/2   tsp. each cayenne pepper and black pepper
1/2   tsp. crushed red pepper flakes
6   cups low sodium chicken broth
1/2   cup tomato paste
1   15 oz. can chopped, stewed tomatoes
1/3   cup finely chopped dry roast peanuts

In large soup pot sprayed with olive oil, cook onion and garlic over medium heat until soft. Add remaining ingredients and heat through; do not boil.

Yield: 12 servings   Count: 2 PRO 1 VEG

Basic Vegetable Soup

5	carrots, peeled and sliced
3	medium celery stalks, sliced
3	large onions, chopped
1	garlic clove, minced
2	28 oz. cans tomato juice
1	small head cabbage, thinly sliced
2	medium parsnips
10	oz. spinach leaves
1/2	cup parsley, chopped
2	chicken bouillon cubes
1	tsp. salt
1/2	tsp. pepper

Cook carrots, celery, onion and garlic in non-stick pan. Add remaining ingredients and 12 cups water. Simmer until vegetables are tender.

Yield: 25 servings   Count: 1 VEG

Beef and Barley Soup

6	celery stalks, diced
1	large onion, diced
4	carrots, thinly sliced
1/2	head red cabbage, sliced
1	lb. beef round, cut in 1/2" cubes
1/2	tsp. salt
2	14.5 oz. cans beef broth

1   14.5 oz. can diced tomato
3/4   cup pearl barley

Brown meat in nonstick pot sprayed with nonstick coating. Add all remaining ingredients and 6 cups water. Reduce heat to simmer for 1 hour. May be frozen for quick meals.

Yield: 8 servings   Count: 3 PRO 1 CHO 2 VEG

Beef and Vegetable Soup

3/4   lb. lean ground beef
1   clove garlic
1/2   tsp. pepper
1/4   tsp. salt
2   13.5 oz. cans beef broth
1   15 oz. can Italian stewed tomatoes
1   cup each sliced carrot and zucchini
1   15 oz. can cannellini beans
2   cups torn spinach leaves

Cook meat with garlic in nonstick pan; drain. Add remaining ingredients, bring to boil and simmer for 10 minutes.

Yield: 4 servings   Count: 3 PRO 1 CHO 2 VEG

Black Bean Soup

1/2	cup onion, chopped
3	cloves garlic, minced
2	15 oz. cans black beans, rinsed & drained
2	tsp. each cumin and oregano
1	tsp. chili powder
1	cup each carrots and mushrooms, sliced
2	15 oz. cans tomato sauce with no added salt
2	14 oz. cans beef broth with no added salt
1	bay leaf
2	Tbsp. lime juice

In large pot sprayed with nonstick spray, sauté onion and garlic until tender. Add remaining ingredients except lime juice. Bring to boil; reduce heat and simmer for 45 minutes. Add lime juice, and simmer another 10 minutes. Discard bay leaf.

Yield: 8 servings   Count: 1 PRO 1 CHO 1 VEG

Black Bean Soup---Quick Version

2	15 oz. cans black beans with no added salt
1/2	cup salsa
1	Tbsp. chili powder
1	16 oz. can chicken broth
1/2	cup (2 oz.) reduced fat cheddar cheese
6	Tbsp. each low fat sour cream and minced green onion

Place beans with liquid in saucepan; partially mash beans with potato masher. Add salsa, chili powder and broth. Bring to boil. Divide into servings and top with remaining ingredients.

Yield: 6 servings   Count: 2 PRO 2 CHO

Butternut Squash Soup

2	Tbsp. olive oil
2	cups chopped onion
2	Tbsp. chopped, seeded jalapeno pepper
1/2 to 1	tsp. curry powder
3	lb. butternut squash
4	cups water
1	tsp. salt
1	cup 1% milk (or soy)
2	Tbsp. dry sherry

Prick squash and microwave until slightly tender, about 7 minutes; cool, then peel and dice, removing seeds. Meanwhile, cook onion in oil until tender; add pepper and curry. Combine all except milk and sherry. Simmer for 30 minutes. Blend squash mixture; add milk and sherry then heat to serve.

Yield: 8 servings   Count: 1 CHO

Cheesy Tomato Soup

2	28 oz. cans whole tomatoes
5	cups chicken broth
3	cups shredded Cheddar cheese
1	6 oz. can tomato paste
1	tsp. each dried parsley and basil
1/2	tsp. dried tarragon
1	pinch dried thyme
	Salt and pepper to taste

In blender, puree tomatoes until smooth. Pour into saucepan. Stir in broth, cheese, and tomato paste. Add seasonings. Simmer 30 minutes, stirring frequently, until cheese is melted and flavors are well-blended.

Yield: 8 servings   Count: 2 PRO 2 VEG 2 FAT

Chicken Soup

4	4 oz. chicken breasts, boneless and skinless
2	cans chicken broth
1	clove garlic, diced
4	small red potatoes, diced
1/2	lb. green beans, cut into 1″ pieces
1/2	cup green onion, sliced
1/2	tsp. each cumin and oregano
1	tsp. chili powder
	Salt and pepper to taste

Microwave chicken breasts until done; dice. Combine with remaining ingredients and simmer until vegetables are tender.

Yield: 4 servings   Count: 3 PRO 1 CHO 1 VEG

Chicken Soup Quick

1	onion, diced
2	carrots, sliced
1	celery stalks, sliced
2	cups green beans
1	14 oz. can chicken broth
1/2	tsp. each thyme, salt and pepper
1/2	cup dry pasta
12	oz. chicken breasts, cooked and thinly sliced

Combine vegetables and broth with 3 cups water; bring to boil. Add seasonings, pasta, and chicken. Cook over medium heat for 10 minutes.

Yield: 4 servings.   Count: 3 PRO 1 CHO 2 VEG

Chicken Tortellini Soup

4   cups vegetable or chicken broth
2-1/2 cups diced cooked chicken
1   cup each sliced celery, carrots, zucchini
1   box frozen chopped spinach
2   cups marinara sauce
1   8 oz. pkg. of prepared tortellini

Combine all ingredients in large pot, except tortellini, and bring to boil. Cover and reduce heat to simmer; cook until vegetables are tender. Add tortellini and simmer until tender, about 10 minutes. Season as desired.

Yield: 6 servings   Count: 3 PRO 1 CHO 1 VEG

Clam Chowder (no milk)

1   potatoes, peeled and diced
1   cup each carrot, celery, and mushrooms, sliced
1/2   cup onion, diced
2   cups soy milk
2   cups clams, solids and liquid
4   slices bacon, cooked and chopped (optional)
        Salt, pepper, garlic to taste

Cook vegetables in a small amount of water until tender. Add remaining ingredients and simmer until heated through.

Yield: 4 servings   Count: 2 PRO 1 CHO 1 VEG

Creamy Tomato Soy Soup

1   10-3/4. oz can tomato soup
1/2   box Mori Nu reduced fat tofu, blended
1-1/4   cup soy milk
1   cup canned diced tomatoes

Combine all ingredients in saucepan. Simmer, stirring frequently.

Yield: 4 servings   Count: 1 PRO 1 CHO

Creamy Zucchini Soup

1   cup chopped onion
2   cloves garlic, minced
10   cups sliced zucchini
1/2   tsp. each salt and pepper
1   tsp. dried tarragon leaves
6   cups chicken broth

Combine all ingredients in large stock pot. Bring to boil; reduce heat and simmer until vegetables are tender. Place 1/3 of mixture at a time in blender and process until smooth. Reheat to serve.

Yield: 10 servings   Count: 1 VEG

Eggplant and Red Pepper Soup

2	red bell peppers
1	eggplant (1-1/2 lb.)
3	cups chicken broth
1-1/2	cup onion, chopped
1/4	cup fresh basil
	Salt and pepper to taste

Cut peppers and eggplant in half; remove seeds from pepper. Place both skin side up on foil-lined baking sheet, and broil for 15 minutes. Seal peppers in zip top bag for 10 minutes. Peel peppers and scoop out eggplant pulp. Discard skins. Combine all ingredients and simmer for 15 minutes. Puree all ingredients until smooth.

Yield: 4 servings   Count: 3 VEG

Fish Chowder

6-7	thick slices bacon
3	cups yellow onion, diced
2	Yukon Gold potatoes
1	baking potato
1	lb. haddock
1	lb. cod
2	cups 1% milk or soy milk
1	cup chicken broth
	Salt and pepper to taste

Fry bacon and drain on paper towel. Sauté onion in bacon fat and set aside. Cut potatoes into cubes and cook with 1 cup chicken broth until tender. Meanwhile, cut fish into bite-sized pieces. When potatoes are cooked, add fish, onions and bacon. When fish flakes, add milk. Bring to boil and simmer 5 minutes. Add salt and pepper to taste.

Yield: 8 servings   Count: 3 PRO 1 VEG

Ganz Family Gazpacho Soup

1	cup or can chopped tomato
1/2	cup each green pepper, celery and cucumber, finely chopped
1/4	cup onion, finely chopped
2	tsp. parsley
1	tsp. chives, optional
2	cloves garlic, minced
2-3	Tbsp. tarragon wine vinegar
2	Tbsp. olive oil
1-1/2	tsp salt, or to taste
1/4	tsp. black pepper, freshly ground
1	Tbsp. Worcestershire sauce
2	cups tomato juice, not from concentrate

Combine all ingredients in glass or stainless bowl. Chill at least 4 hours. Remove from refrigerator 1 hour before serving.

Yield: 6 servings   Count: 1-1/2 VEG

Gazpacho Andaluz

8	ripe tomatoes
1	each onion, cucumber, and green pepper
1	clove garlic
4	oz. French bread
1/3	cup salad oil
1/3	cup red wine vinegar
1	Tbsp. salt

Soak bread in water to soften. Put all ingredients in blender or food processor and blend to desired consistency. Serve cold.

Yield: 8 servings   Count: 1 VEG 1/2 CHO 2 FAT
                                       1 VEG (omitting bread and oil)

Gazpacho with Garlic

1	cup yellow pepper, chopped
1	cucumber, peeled and seeded, chopped
1/4	cup sherry vinegar
1	tsp. olive oil
1/2	tsp. each salt and pepper
2-1/4	lb. plum tomatoes, halved
6	garlic cloves
4	ice cubes

Combine all ingredients in blender and process until smooth. Cover and chill.

Yield: 6 servings   Count: 2 VEG

Gumbo with Shrimp or Chicken

4	Tbsp. olive oil, divided
1	each red onion, garlic clove and green pepper
4	stalk celery
4	Tbsp. flour
1	14 oz. can ready-cut tomatoes
2	14 oz. cans chicken broth
1/2	tsp. each black, white and red pepper
1/2	tsp. each thyme and oregano
1	bay leaf
1/2	lb. frozen okra, sliced
1	lb. cooked shrimp or cooked and diced chicken breast

Sauté vegetables in 2 Tbsp. oil; remove vegetables; add remaining oil. Add flour and stir; cook until light golden brown. Gradually add chicken broth, 1/2 cup water and tomatoes, stirring constantly; add seasonings and simmer 15 minutes. Add okra and shrimp and heat another 15 minutes.

Yield: 6 servings   Count: 3 PRO 2 VEG

Italian Sausage Soup

16   oz. sweet Italian turkey sausage
3   cups chicken broth
2   15 oz. cans Italian seasoned diced tomatoes
1/2   cup uncooked small shell pasta
8   oz. baby spinach leaves

In large pot, slice sausage and cook over medium heat until browned, about 5 minutes. Drain and return to pot. Add broth, tomatoes, and pasta, and bring to boil over high heat. Cover, reduce heat, and simmer for 10 minutes or until pasta is tender. Remove from heat; stir in spinach.

Yield: 4 servings   Count: 3 PRO 3 VEG

Mu Shu Pork Soup

4   oz. lean pork loin, cut in 1/4″ by 1″ pieces
2   Tbsp. hoisin sauce
1/4   cup dry sherry (optional)
1/2   tsp. sesame oil
1   6" flour tortilla
1   tsp. hoisin sauce
1-1/2 clove garlic, minced
1   large carrot, shredded
1-1/2 cups cabbage, shredded
1/2   cup mushrooms, sliced
1-1/2 Tbsp cornstarch
5   cups low salt chicken broth

1	Tbsp. each soy sauce and Worcestershire sauce
1	Tbsp. each grated ginger and lemon juice
1/4	cup diced red pepper
2	scallions, chopped

Marinate pork with 2 Tbsp. hoisin, 1 Tbsp sherry, and sesame oil for 1 hour.

Spread tortilla with 1 tsp. hoisin sauce. Cut into 1/8″ strip. Bake at 300 degrees for 30 minutes or until crispy. Set aside.

Drain marinade from pork. Do not reuse. Spray a large nonstick pan with nonstick spray. Over medium heat, sauté drained pork for 2 to 3 minutes. Set aside. Add garlic, carrot, and cabbage and sauté for 4 minutes; add a few tsp. water as needed. Add remaining ingredients and bring to boil. Return pork and scallions. Top with tortilla strips to serve.

Yield: 4 servings   Count: 1 PRO 1/2 CHO 1 VEG

Potato Soup

2	Tbsp. soft tub margarine
1	medium onion, chopped
1	stalk celery, chopped
1	carrot, chopped
2	cloves garlic, minced
1-1/4	lb. yellow potatoes, peeled and cubed
1	14 oz. can chicken broth
3/4	tsp. salt
1/4	tsp. pepper

Melt margarine; add next three ingredients and cook until tender. Add remaining ingredients and 3 cups water. Simmer until potatoes are tender. Blend in processor until smooth. Heat through to serve.

Yield: 8 servings   Count: 1 CHO

Pumpkin Soup

1	14 oz. can vegetable broth
1	large onion
2	carrots, diced
1/3	tsp. salt
1/8	tsp. pepper
2	cups nonfat or soy milk
1	tsp. cinnamon
1	16 oz. can canned pumpkin
1	box Mori Nu firm tofu (12.3 oz.), cubed

Combine broth, carrots, onion, salt and pepper. Simmer uncovered for 15 minutes or until vegetables are soft. Add remaining ingredients and simmer for 10 minutes.

Yield: 4 servings   Count: 1 CHO 1 PRO 1 VEG

Red Pepper Soup from Rubye Schneider

6	red peppers
1	large carrot
1	stalk celery
1	medium onion
3-4	garlic cloves
	Salt and pepper to taste
1/2	cup rice, uncooked
1	large and 1 small can chicken broth
1/2	tsp. each cumin and thyme

Sauté vegetables until tender. Add remaining ingredients and simmer for 30 minutes. Process in blender until smooth.

Yield: 8 servings   Count: 1 VEG

Sausage and Kale Soup

12	oz. turkey kielbasa, sliced
1	large onion, chopped
1	large garlic clove, chopped
1	tsp. olive oil
1	10 oz. pkg. frozen kale
2	14 oz. cans reduced sodium chicken broth
4	cups water
2	carrots, sliced
1	tsp. dried leaf marjoram, crumbled
1/2	tsp. salt
1/8	tsp. pepper
1/2	cup uncooked long grain rice

Sauté kielbasa, onion, and garlic in oil in large pot until tender, about 10 minutes. Add remaining ingredients (except rice) and bring to boil. Lower heat and simmer for 15 minutes; add rice and simmer for another 15 minutes or until rice is tender.

Yield: 4 servings   Count: 3 PRO 1 CHO 2 VEG

Squash and Apple Soup

6	cups chicken broth, divided
1	small butternut squash, peeled and cubed
1	large sweet potato, peeled and cubed
2	cups onion, diced
2	Granny Smith apples, peeled and diced
4	tsp. Butter
1	Tbsp. Flour

Salt and pepper to taste

Combine 5 cups broth, squash, and potato in large pot; bring to boil. Cover, reduce heat and simmer until vegetables are tender. With slotted spoon remove vegetables and blend until smooth; add back to broth. In microwave-proof dish cook 1 tsp. butter, apples and onion until tender; add to squash mixture. Melt remaining 3 tsp. butter and add flour; cook for 5 minutes or until golden brown, stirring constantly with a whisk. Gradually add 1 cup broth and cook for 3 minutes or until slightly thickened. Add thickened broth to remaining mixture; heat over medium heat until heated through; season to taste.

Yield: 10 servings   Count: 1 CHO

Sweet and Sour Vegetable Soup

12   cups chicken broth
2   14.5 oz. cans diced tomato
2   cups sliced carrots
1-1/2   cups each onion and celery, diced
6   cups cabbage, coarsely chopped
1   cup cider vinegar
1/2   cup Splenda
        Salt and pepper to taste

Pour broth and tomatoes into large pot. Add carrots and simmer 10 minutes. Add remaining ingredients and simmer until vegetables are tender.

Yield: 16 servings   Count: 1 VEG

Tomato Basil Soup from Margaret Johnson

8- 10   ripe tomatoes, peeled, seeded and chopped
1   cups tomato juice
1   cup chicken broth
14   fresh basil leaves
1   cup evaporated skim milk
1   4 oz. package Butter Buds

Simmer tomatoes, juice, and broth for 30 minutes. Puree tomato mixture with basil and Butter Buds; return to pan, add milk; heat until hot and thickened.

Yield: 8 servings   Count: 1 VEG

Vegetable Soup—version 1

1/2   lb. carrot, sliced
1/4   lb. turnip, cubed and peeled
1/2   lb. red potato, cubed and peeled
1/2   cup celery, chopped
3/4   cup water
1   16 oz. box chicken broth
1/2   tsp. sage
       Salt and pepper to taste

Combine all vegetables, water, and broth. Cover and bring to boil. Simmer until vegetables are tender; add seasonings. Puree in blender until smooth; reheat to serve.

Yield: 4 servings   Count: 1 VEG 1/2 CHO

Vegetable Soup –version 2

1	Tbsp. olive oil
2- 1/2	cup chopped onion
1	cup chopped carrot
5	plum tomatoes, halved
1	green pepper, chopped
3	clove garlic, sliced
4	cup vegetable broth
1	cup potato, peeled and diced
1	tsp. each oregano and basil
1	28 oz. can tomatoes
	Salt and pepper to taste

Preheat oven to 425 degrees. Combine first six ingredients in plastic bag; shake to coat. Remove from bag onto a baking sheet. Bake for 30 minutes or until tender. Combine remaining ingredients and simmer until potato is tender; add vegetables. Blend mixture until smooth. Heat to serve. Add salt and pepper to taste.

Yield: 10 servings   Count: 2 VEG

Side Dishes

Asparagus and Ham Appetizer

24	asparagus spears
2	large sheets phyllo dough, thawed
12	thin slices ham (6 oz.)
12	thin slices cheese (6 oz.)
2	Tbsp. butter, melted

Steam asparagus spears for 3 minutes; set aside. Lay one sheet of phyllo dough on cutting board; brush with butter; top with next sheet and repeat. Cut sheets into 12 rectangles. To assemble, place ham and cheese slice on each rectangle; place 2 asparagus spears on top; roll up and place on baking sheet; brush with remaining butter. Bake at 350 degrees for 10 minutes. Serve warm.

Yield: 12 servings   Count: 1 PRO 1/2 VEG

Bread Dressing

4	cups bread cubes
1/2	cup chopped celery
1/4	cup chopped onion
1	Tbsp. chopped fresh parsley leaves
1/2	clove garlic, minced
1/4	cup hot water
1/4	tsp. each black pepper, sage, marjoram, thyme, and basil

Combine all ingredients; pour into lightly oiled casserole dish. Bake at 350 degrees for 30 minutes.

Yield: 4 servings   Count: 1 CHO

Chicken Tofu Dip

1   box Mori Nu reduced fat tofu
1   Tbsp. lemon juice
1   Tbsp. each taco seasoning and minced onion
1   tsp. garlic powder
1   3-1/2 oz. can chicken

Mix tofu, garlic powder, taco seasoning and lemon juice in blender until creamy; stir in chicken and onion. Chill.

Yield: 6 servings   Count: 1 PRO

Cucumbers Vinaigrette

3   cucumbers, peeled, halved lengthwise, seeded and thinly sliced (about 3-1/2 cups)
1/2   cup vertically sliced red onion
1   tsp. each dried basil and parsley
2   Tbsp. red wine vinegar
1   Tbsp. olive oil
2-1/2 tsp. Dijon mustard
1/4   tsp. salt

Place cucumbers and onion in bowl. Combine basil and remaining ingredients; pour over cucumber mixture. Toss gently. Cover and chill.

Yield: 6 servings   Count: 1 VEG

Curried Dip

1	cup nonfat plain yogurt
1/4	cup chutney
1/2	tsp. curry powder
1/4	tsp. salt

Combine all ingredients and chill.

Yield: 20 servings   Count: FREE

Greek Garlic Dip

2	large potatoes, peeled
5- 6	garlic cloves crushed
1	cup parsley leaves
1/2	cup olive oil
3	Tbsp. vinegar
	Salt and pepper

Boil potatoes until tender, dice. Add half of oil and the vinegar to a blender with potato and garlic. Blend until smooth, adding more oil as needed; season to taste.

Yield: 2 cups   Count: 1 Tbsp. = FREE
                        1/4 cup = 1/2 CHO

Low Fat Layered Ranchero Dip

1	28 oz. can pinto beans, drained and mashed
1/2	tsp. cumin
1/3	cup each nonfat plain yogurt, sour cream, and mayonnaise
1	Tbsp. taco seasoning
1	tsp. taco seasoning
4	oz. diced green chilies
3	oz. nonfat cheddar cheese
1/4	cup diced green onion
2	cups diced tomato

Combine beans, cumin, and half of the chilies and spread in 10˝ pan. Combine yogurt, sour cream, and mayonnaise with taco seasoning. Spread over beans. Sprinkle with remaining ingredients.

Yield: 14 servings   Count: 1 PRO 1 CHO

Salsa Verde Dip

1/2	cup salsa verde
1/2	cup low fat cottage cheese.

Combine ingredients and chill.

Yield: 16 servings   Count: FREE

Shrimp Dip

1/3   cup fat free sour cream or Tofutti Sour Supreme
8   oz. fat-free cream cheese or soy substitute
1/2   cup each celery and onion, chopped
2   Tbsp. lemon juice
1/4   tsp. each salt and pepper
3/4   lb. cooked salad shrimp
Combine all ingredients and chill.

Yield: 12 servings   Count: 1 PRO

Spinach and Artichoke Dip

2   cups part-skim mozzarella cheese, shredded, divided
1/2   cup fat-free sour cream
1/4   cup fresh Parmesan cheese, grated, divided
1/4   tsp. black pepper
3   cloves garlic, crushed
1   can artichoke hearts, drained and chopped
8   oz. reduced fat cream cheese, softened
8   oz. fat-free cream cheese, softened
1/2   10 oz. pkg. frozen chopped spinach, thawed, drained, and squeezed dry

Combine 1-1/2 cups of the mozzarella, sour cream, 2 Tbsp. of the Parmesan and remaining ingredients; stir until well blended. Spoon into 1-1/2 qt. baking dish. Top with 1/2 cup mozzarella and 2 Tbsp. Parmesan. Bake at 350 degrees for 30 minutes.

Yield: 20 servings   Count: 1 PRO 1 VEG

Sarah's Onion Dip

6   oz. Tofutti Better Than Sour Cream
4   oz. Tofutti Better Than Cream Cheese
1-1/2 oz. onion soup mix, dry
1   12.3 oz. box Mori Nu Lite Silken Tofu
Blend all ingredients together and chill.

Yield: 6 servings.   Count: 1/2 CHO 1 PRO

Spinach Dip

1   tsp. olive oil
3   garlic cloves , chopped
1/4   tsp. salt
1   10 oz. package fresh spinach
1/2   cup basil leaves
3   oz. reduced fat cream cheese, softened
1/8   tsp. pepper
1/3   cup plain fat-free yogurt
1/4   cup Parmesan cheese, grated
Heat oil in large skillet over medium heat. Add garlic and sauté for 1 minute. Add salt and spinach; sauté 3 minutes or until spinach wilts. Place spinach in colander and press out water. Place spinach, basil, pepper, and cream cheese in food processor or mixer and blend until smooth. Stir in yogurt and Parmesan. Chill.

Yield: 8 servings   Count: 1/2 VEG 1/2 PRO

Tex-Mex Black Bean Dip

1	15 oz. can black beans, drained
1	tsp. olive oil
1/2	cup onion, chopped
2	garlic cloves, minced
1/4	cup tomato, diced
1/3	cup mild picante sauce
1/2	tsp. cumin
1/3	tsp. chili powder
1/3	cup shredded low fat jack cheese
1/4	cup cilantro, chopped
1	Tbsp. fresh lime juice

Mash beans until chunky; set aside. Heat oil and add onion and garlic; sauté about 4 minutes until tender. Add next four ingredients (tomato, picante sauce, cumin and chili powder) and cook 5 minutes. Combine with beans. Sprinkle with cheese, cilantro, and lime juice to serve.

Yield: 16 servings   Count: 1/3 CHO

Vegetables

Asparagus Roasted

1-1/2 lb. asparagus
1   clove garlic, minced
2   tsp. olive oil
1/2   tsp. salt
1/4   tsp. each thyme and pepper

Heat oven to 400 degrees. Break off tough ends of asparagus; wash and cut diagonally into 2 inch sections. Put all ingredients in plastic bag and shake to coat asparagus. Spread in baking dish and bake for 20 minutes; stir after 10 minutes.

Yield: 6 servings   Count: 1 VEG

Bean and Sausage Stew

1   15 oz. can kidney beans, drained
1   lb. Italian turkey sausage, no casing
1   medium onion, chopped
2   clove garlic, minced
1   cup carrot, chopped
1/2   cup celery, chopped
1   15 oz. can chicken broth
1   15 oz. can diced tomato
1   medium tomato, peeled and chopped
1   tsp. each basil and oregano
1   cup pasta of choice, dry
1   10 oz. pkg. frozen chopped spinach

Sauté sausage, onion, and garlic; drain. Add next six ingredients; bring to boil, cover and simmer for 15 minutes. Stir in pasta; bring to boil; reduce heat; add beans and spinach. Cover and simmer for 15 minutes or until pasta is tender.

Yield: 10 servings   Count: 2 PRO 1 CHO 1 VEG

Braised Red Cabbage

2   Tbsp. butter or margarine
1/2   red onion, diced
1   head red cabbage, quartered, cored, sliced 1/4"
1   apple, peeled and diced
2   Tbsp. brown sugar
3   Tbsp. cider or wine vinegar
1   tsp. salt
1/4   tsp. pepper

Melt butter; add onion and cook until tender. Add cabbage and stir until slightly wilted. Add remaining ingredients and 1/2 cup water; simmer for 1 hour, stirring occasionally.

Yield: 8 servings   Count 2 VEG

Collards with Bacon

2   slices bacon, chopped
1/2   sweet onion, chopped
1   lb. collard greens; washed
1/2   tsp. salt
1/4   tsp. pepper

Cook bacon until crisp; drain on paper towel. Add onion to drippings and cook until tender. Discard stems of greens and chop leaves. Add to onions with salt and pepper. Cook, stirring frequently, about 5 minutes until tender. Add bacon pieces.

Yield: 4 servings   Count: 1 VEG

Corn Casserole

3   Tbsp. butter, softened
3   large egg whites
8   oz. fat-free cream cheese
1/2   cup each chopped onion and red pepper
1   15 oz. can whole kernel corn, drained
1   14 oz. can cream-style corn
1   8 oz. package corn muffin mix

Preheat oven to 375 degrees. Combine first three ingredients in large bowl, stirring with whisk until smooth. Stir in onion, pepper, and both types of corn. Mix well. Add muffin mix and stir until well combined. Pour into 11 by 7 inch baking dish coated with cooking spray. Bake for 50 minutes or until pick inserted in center comes out clean.

Yield: 18 servings   Count: 1 CHO 1/2 PRO

Green Bean Casserole

1	lb. green beans
8	oz. fresh mushrooms, sliced
1	bunch green onion, sliced
1	cup milk or soy milk
2	Tbsp. flour; salt and pepper to taste
2	Tbsp. margarine
3	Tbsp. Nutlettes

Steam green beans; set aside. Sauté mushrooms and green beans in margarine. Gradually add flour to milk; cook over low heat, stirring constantly, until thickened. Combine all ingredients and place in casserole dish sprayed with non-stick spray; top with Nutlettes. Bake for 30 minutes at 300 degrees.

Yield: 8 servings   Count: 1 VEG

Low-Carb Mashed Potato

1	head cauliflower, steamed
2	Tbsp. instant mashed potato granules
3	Tbsp. sheep's milk Romano cheese

Blend all ingredients together. Heat to serve.

Yield: 4 servings   Count: 2 VEG

Ratatouille

1	cup onion, sliced
1	cup each red and green pepper strips
10	garlic cloves, minced
1/4	cup fresh basil, chopped
1/4	tsp. each salt and pepper
2	cup zucchini, sliced
3	medium tomatoes, sliced
1	small eggplant, peeled and sliced

Combine onion, peppers, and garlic and cook in micro-wave for 4 minutes; set aside. Spray a 13 by 9 inch pan with nonstick spray. Layer half of zucchini, tomato, and eggplant, then top with half the onion mix. Repeat. Cover and bake at 350 degrees for 40 minutes.

Yield: 8 servings   Count: 2 VEG

Red Cabbage with Apple

2	Tbsp. oil
2	medium red onions, sliced
1	head red cabbage, cored and sliced 1/4-inch thick
1	golden delicious apple, cored and diced
1	Tbsp. sugar
1-1/2	tsp. salt
3	Tbsp. cider vinegar

Heat oil in large sauce pan. Add onion and cook 10 to 12 minutes or until tender and lightly browned. Gradually add cabbage, stirring until wilted, about 6 minutes. Add apple, sugar, and salt and cook 5 minutes longer. Stir in vinegar.

Yield: 9 servings   Count: 2 VEG

Rosemary Potatoes

2-1/2	lb. assorted small potatoes (red, white, purple, golden)
3	Tbsp. olive oil
1	Tbsp. fresh rosemary, chopped
3/4	tsp. salt
1/4	tsp. black pepper

Preheat oven to 425 degrees. Place potatoes in roasting pan and toss with remaining ingredients. Roast for 30 to 40 minutes, turning occasionally until golden and fork tender.

Yield: 10 servings.   Count: 1 CHO

Sweet 'n Sour Red Cabbage

2   Tbsp. butter or margarine

1/2   red onion, diced

1   head red cabbage, quartered, cored, and sliced 1/4" thick

1   apple, peeled and diced

2   Tbsp. brown sugar

3   Tbsp. cider or wine vinegar

1   tsp. salt

1/4   tsp. pepper

Melt margarine; add onion and cook until tender. Add cabbage and stir until slightly wilted. Add remaining ingredients and 1/2 cup water; simmer for 1 hour, stirring occasionally.

Yield: 8 servings   Count: 2 VEG

Squash Sauté

3/4   lb. zucchini, sliced

3/4   lb. yellow summer squash, sliced

3   green onions, sliced

1   Tbsp. margarine or butter

1/2   tsp. salt

1/8   tsp. pepper

Combine all ingredients in microwave dish. Cook covered on high heat for 8 to 10 minutes; stir halfway through cooking.

Yield: 4 servings   Count: 1 VEG

Squash Cakes

4	cups shredded zucchini squash (8 to 10)
3/4	cup crushed saltine crackers
1	egg or 1/4 cup egg substitute
	Seasoning to taste: salt, pepper, and garlic

Combine all ingredients in bowl. Cook about 1/4 cup batter at a time in frying pan coated lightly with olive oil.

Yield: 8 servings   Count: 1/2 CHO 1 VEG

Thai Broccoli

1	bunch broccoli, cut into florets
2	Tbsp. low sodium soy sauce
1	Tbsp. vegetable oil
1	tsp. lime peel

Combine all ingredients and cook covered in microwave on high for 7 to 10 minutes or until tender. Garnish with cilantro or parsley and sliced radishes.

Yield: 4 servings   Count: 1 VEG

Vegetable Chili from Sandy Ward

4	medium onions, chopped
4	medium carrots, cut in 1/2″ pieces
2	Tbsp. garlic, minced
2	Tbsp. each chili powder and cumin
1/2	lb. red potato, cut in 1/2″ cubes

1   each red, green, and yellow bell peppers, seeded and cut into 1/2″ pieces

2   28 oz. cans peeled tomatoes

1   Tbsp. tomato paste

1   Tbsp. brown sugar

2   tsp. oregano

1   tsp. fennel

2   each yellow and zucchini squash, cut into 1/2″ cubes

1/2   cup parsley

2   Tbsp. lemon juice

Combine all ingredients in large pot and bring to boil; turn down heat and simmer until vegetables are tender.

Yield: 10 servings   Count: 2 VEG

Vegetable Packets Grilled

4   small potatoes, quartered

4   each onion slices and green pepper rings

4   plum tomatoes, quartered

1   cup carrot, thinly sliced

4   Tbsp. reduced calorie margarine

1/4   tsp. each salt and pepper

Divide ingredients into four portions and wrap each in aluminum foil. Grill for 15 minutes; turn and cook 10 minutes.

Yield: 4 servings   Count: 1 VEG 1 CHO

Vegetable Stew from Kelly

2	each onion, carrot, red pepper, tomato, celery rib
1	cup mushrooms
1	can wax bean, drained
1	10 oz. pkg. frozen green beans
6	oz. can tomato paste
1	Tbsp. sugar
1	tsp. salt

Slice all vegetables. Combine all ingredients, adding 1 cup water. Cover and simmer for 20 minutes.

Yield: 8 servings   Count: 2 VEG

Vegetable Stew

2	Tbsp. olive oil
1	cup red onion
2	cups green pepper, chopped
2	cloves garlic, minced
1	cup mushrooms, sliced and fresh parsley
1	small eggplant
1	28 oz. can crushed tomatoes
1/2	cup kalamata olives
1	15 oz. can garbanzo beans
1	Tbsp. rosemary

Sauteé onion in oil. Add remaining ingredients and simmer until vegetables are tender.

Yield: 6 servings.   Count: 1 CHO 4 VEG

White Italian Beans

1-1/2 Tbsp. olive oil
1   cup finely chopped onion
1/8   tsp. crushed red pepper
4   garlic cloves, minced
1   bay leaf
1   Tbsp. Water
1   16 oz. can Great Northern or navy beans, rinsed and drained
2   tsp. white vinegar
1/4   tsp. salt
1/8   tsp. black pepper

Heat oil in large nonstick skillet over medium heat. Add onion and sauteé 3 minutes; add next three ingredients and cook for additional 3 minutes. Stir in water and beans. Cook 3 minutes or until heated. Add remaining ingredients. Discard bay leaf.

Yield: 4 servings   Count: 1 PRO 1 CHO

Entreées

Baked Fish Fillets

1	lb. fish fillet
1	Tbsp. lemon juice
1/4	tsp. each salt and onion powder
2	tsp. light mayonnaise
2	Tbsp. each bread crumbs and parsley

Place fish in baking dish coated with nonstick spray. Combine juice through mayonnaise and spread on fish. Sprinkle with crumbs and parsley. Bake at 400 degrees for 20 to 25 minutes or until fish flakes easily.

Yield: 4 servings   Count: 3 PRO

Balsamic Chicken with Grapes and Almonds

4	4 oz. chicken breasts, boneless and skinless
1/2	tsp. salt
1/8	tsp. pepper
2	tsp. olive oil
1	cup seedless red grapes, halved
1/2	cup fat-free low sodium chicken broth
2	Tbsp. balsamic vinegar
1	Tbsp. brown sugar
1/4	cup sliced almonds

Heat oil over medium heat. Add chicken and sprinkle with salt and pepper. Sauté until golden brown (about 3 minutes per side). Remove chicken. Add remaining ingredients except almonds. Bring mixture to boil; cook until about 1 cup remains (approx. 6 minutes). Return chicken to pan and cook 3 minutes or until done, turning to coat. Sprinkle with almonds to serve.

Yield: 4 servings   Count: 3 PRO 1/2 CHO

Basil Mushroom Burgers from Sandy Cohen

1/2	onion, finely chopped
3	Tbsp. nonfat milk
1	egg
2	Tbsp. fresh basil, chopped (1 tsp. dry)
2	tsp. Dijon mustard
1/4	tsp. each salt and pepper
1/4	cup dry bread crumbs
1-1/4	lb. ground turkey

Combine all ingredients. Form into patties and cook in lightly greased skillet about 5 minutes per side or until juices run clear.

Yield: 5 patties   Count: 3 PRO

Butternut Chili

1	lb. ground turkey or beef
1	cup each chopped onion and bell pepper
3	large tomatoes, chopped
1	small butternut squash, peeled and chopped
3	cups water
1	tsp. each oregano, cumin and chili powder
2	cloves garlic, minced

Brown meat and stir to crumble; drain. Add remaining ingredients and bring to boil. Reduce heat and simmer for 20 minutes or until squash is tender.

Yield: 4 servings   Count: 3 PRO 1 CHO 2 VEG

Beef Empanadas

1	cup each finely chopped red potato and onion
1	cup beef broth
1/4	tsp. each salt, ground cumin, allspice, pepper
1/2	lb. top sirloin, trimmed and diced
1	garlic clove, minced
1	Tbsp. finely chopped cilantro
1	Tbsp. each cornstarch and cold water
36	won ton wrappers

Combine ingredients through cilantro in saucepan. Bring to boil, simmer until potato is done (about 8 minutes). Remove from heat and cool. Preheat oven to 400 degrees and place two baking sheets in oven for about 10 minutes. Drain meat mixture and blend until finely chopped. Take one won ton wrapper at a time, and place 1 Tbsp. meat mix in center. Moisten edges with cornstarch mixture; bring opposite corners together to form triangle; seal edges. Coat baking sheets with cooking spray, place empanadas in a single layer; coat with cooking spray. Bake 8 minutes or until golden, turning once.

Yield: 36   Count: 3 = 1/2 CHO 1/2 PRO

Chard and Bean Frittata

7   large egg whites, lightly beaten
2   large eggs, lightly beaten
1/2   tsp. salt
1/4   tsp. black pepper
1   16 oz. can white beans, rinsed and drained
1   tsp. olive oil
2   cups torn Swiss chard or spinach
1-1/2   cup chopped onion

Heat oil in large non-stick skillet. Add chard and onion and cook until chard is limp. Combine egg whites, eggs, beans and seasonings and pour over chard mixture. Reduce heat to low and cook for 10 minutes or until almost set. Wrap handle of pan with foil and broil until top is brown.

Yield: 4 servings   Count: 2 PRO 1 CHO 1 VEG

Chicken and Seafood Casserole from Mary Reese

1	pkg. soy twist noodles, cooked and drained
6	oz. each steamed scallops and shrimp
12	oz. cooked chicken breast, diced
1	shallot, thinly sliced
1	15 oz. can diced tomato
1	jar artichoke hearts in water, drained
1/2	cup white wine vinegar
	Seasoning salt and pepper to taste
	Sliced green onion tops for garnish

Combine all ingredients. May be served hot or cold.

Yield: 8 servings   Count: 3 PRO 1 CHO 1 VEG

Chicken Adobo from Cody Lee's family—a favorite of three boys

2	lb. chicken, boneless breasts or thighs
1/4	cup vinegar
1/4	cup soy sauce
2	cloves garlic, crushed
1/2	tsp. black peppercorns
1	bay leaf

Combine all ingredients in a large pot. Cover and marinate for 1 to 3 hours. Bring to a boil, then lower heat, cover, and simmer for 30 minutes, stirring occasionally. Uncover and simmer until sauce is reduced and thickened and chicken is tender, about 20 minutes.

Yield: 8 servings   Count: 3 PRO

Chicken and Artichokes

1	Tbsp. olive oil
1	lb. chicken tenders
1/4	tsp. each salt and pepper
1	garlic clove, crushed
1/2	cup chicken broth
1	tsp. cornstarch
1	14 oz. can artichoke hearts, rinsed, drained
1	pt. cherry tomatoes

Heat oil; add chicken, salt and pepper. Cook until lightly browned. Mix garlic, broth and cornstarch. Add to chicken with vegetables, and heat to boiling; cook for 1 minute.

Yield: 4 servings   Count: 3 PRO 1 VEG

Chicken and Barley

1	tsp. cumin
3/4	tsp. chili powder
1/2	tsp. each salt and cinnamon
1/4	tsp. garlic powder
1/8	tsp. pepper
6	chicken breasts, boneless
3/4	cup chopped onion
1/2	cup chopped red bell pepper
1	cup chicken broth
1/2	cup pearl barley
1	14.5 oz. can diced tomato

Combine spices in plastic bag; add chicken and shake to coat. Brown in nonstick pan coated with nonstick spray. Add remaining ingredients. Bring to boil, cover, and simmer for 50 minutes.

Yield: 6 servings   Count: 3 PRO 1 CHO

Chicken Cacciatore from Sandy Tompkins

6	chicken breasts, boneless and skinless
2	large cans marinara sauce
1	can chicken broth
1	jar marinated mushrooms
1	jar pesto (dried tomato and basil)
1	each green, yellow, and red peppers
2	cloves garlic, minced

Brown chicken, garlic, and peppers. Add remaining ingredients and simmer for 4 hours. This also is well-suited for a crock pot.

Yield: 6 servings   Count: 3 PRO 1 VEG

Chicken Cordon Bleu

1	Tbsp. margarine
4	boneless and skinless chicken breasts (1 lb.)
1/2	cup chicken broth
2	Tbsp. balsamic vinegar
1/8	tsp. pepper
4	thin slices each cooked ham and mozzarella cheese
1	bag pre-washed spinach, steamed

Melt margarine in large skillet; add chicken and cook until golden brown about six minutes. Turn over; cover and cook on medium heat for six minutes or until juices run clear. Add chicken broth, vinegar and pepper; cook uncovered for one minute. Remove skillet from heat; top each chicken breast with a slice of ham and cheese. Cover until cheese melts (about 3 minutes). Arrange spinach on plates. Top with chicken breast; drizzle with sauce.

Yield: 4 servings   Count: 4 PRO 1 VEG

Chicken in Mustard Sauce

6	4 oz. chicken breasts, boneless and skinless
1/2	tsp. each salt and pepper
1	Tbsp. canola or olive oil
1	cup chopped onion
1	Tbsp. flour
1-1/2	cup water
1	Tbsp. Dijon mustard
1-1/2	tsp. dry mustard

1 Tbsp. chopped fresh parsley

Heat oil in large skillet over medium high heat. Add chicken and sauté for 2 minutes per side; sprinkle with salt and pepper. Add the onion and continue cooking for 1 minute. Sprinkle the flour on both sides of chicken pieces. Cook for 1 minute to brown flour. Add the water and stir to loosen any solidified pieces. Bring the mixture to a boil, reduce heat to low, and cook for 2 minutes. Remove chicken to serving platter and keep warm in 180-degree oven while you finish the sauce.

Bring the skillet mixture to boil and add the mustards, stirring with a whisk. Return chicken and heat gently (do not boil) until heated through. Arrange on platter and sprinkle with parsley.

Yield: 6 servings   Count: 3 PRO

Chicken Pasta

2	3 oz. cooked chicken sausages, sliced
1	onion, sliced
1	tomato, chopped
1	garlic clove, minced
1	Tbsp. water
1	cup water
1/8	tsp. each salt and pepper
1	cup broccoli florets
1/2	cup each red and yellow pepper, sliced
1	cup (2 oz. dry) cooked pasta
2	tsp. fresh basil, chopped

Coat large skillet with nonstick spray. Stir-fry sausage slices until brown; set aside. Re-coat skillet and stir-fry vegetables. Sprinkle with flour. Add water, salt and pepper. Cover and reduce heat, simmering for about 10 minutes. Add sausage and pasta; heat through; sprinkle with basil.

Yield: 2 servings.   Count: 3 PRO 4 VEG 1 CHO

Chicken and Rice Casserole from Sandy Ward

6   4 oz. chicken breasts, boneless and skinless
1   28 oz. can baked beans
1   14.5 oz. can stewed tomatoes
1-1/2 cups water
1/2   cup uncooked rice
1   tsp. chili powder
1/2   tsp. garlic salt
1   Tbsp. vegetable oil

Mix chili powder and garlic salt; sprinkle over chicken. Brown chicken in oil. Combine chicken and remaining ingredients in 3-quart baking dish, sprayed with nonstick spray. Cover and bake at 400 degrees for 45 minutes.

Yield: 6 servings   Count: 3 PRO 2-1/2 CHO

Chicken Quesadilla

8   oz. pre-cooked chicken breast, diced
8   oz. sliced mushrooms
4   low-carb whole wheat tortillas or 4 fajita-size tortillas
1/2   cup chopped onion
1   jalapeno pepper, seeded and chopped
4   oz. shredded Mexican cheese blend
1   tsp. olive oil
1   tsp. cumin
1/4   tsp. each salt and pepper

Heat oil in non-stick skillet; add onion, pepper, cumin, salt and pepper and sauté 5 minutes; add chicken and heat thru. Set mixture aside; wipe pan with paper towel, then heat at medium setting. Sprinkle tortillas with cheese; add 1/4 mushroom mixture to each. Fold tortilla in half. Cook 2 minutes per side or until light brown and cheese is melted.

Yield: 4 servings   Count: 3 PRO 1 CHO

Chicken Salsa

4   4 oz. boneless and skinless chicken breasts
1   cup salsa
1/2   cup green onion, sliced
1/2   cup mushrooms, sliced
3   cups shredded cabbage

Heat oven to 350 degrees. Spray 11 by 7 inch pan with nonstick spray. Spread cabbage, onions, and mushrooms on bottom of pan. Top with chicken breasts, then top all with salsa. Cover and bake for 30 minutes; uncover and bake additional 10 minutes or until chicken is done and juices run clear when pierced with fork.

Yield: 4 servings   Count: 3 PRO 2 VEG

Chicken Sticks

1/4	cup chopped onion
1/4	cup tofu
1/8	tsp. ginger
1/4	tsp. each salt and pepper
1/4	tsp. cumin
1	garlic clove
6	4 oz. chicken breasts

Place all ingredients except chicken in blender and process until smooth. Combine tofu mix and chicken in resealable plastic bag and marinate in refrigerator for 2 hours. Remove chicken and discard marinade. Thread chicken onto wooden skewers. Broil 6 minutes per side or until chicken is done.

Yield: 6 servings   Count: 3 PRO 1/2 FAT

Chicken Strips from the Raymond Family

4	4 oz. chicken breast halves, skinless and boneless
1	large egg
1	Tbsp. cornstarch
2	tsp. soy sauce
1/2	cup sesame seeds
1/4	cup fine breadcrumbs
½	tsp. garlic powder
3	Tbsp. margarine, melted

Cut chicken into strips. Dip chicken into the combined egg, cornstarch and soy sauce. Let sit 15 minutes. Combine sesame seeds, breadcrumbs and garlic powder in large re-sealable bag; add chicken and shake until coated. Place on lightly greased baking sheet and drizzle with melted margarine. Broil for 5 minutes per side, until golden.

Dipping sauce: Combine 2 Tbsp. mustard and 1 Tbsp. mayonnaise.

Yield: 5 servings   Count: 3 PRO 1/2 CHO

Chicken Vegetable Dish

6	chicken thighs, boneless and skinless
	Flour for coating chicken
4	zucchini squash, sliced
1	red onion
1	red pepper, diced
1	can artichoke hearts
1	14 oz. can stewed tomatoes
1	14 oz. can crushed tomatoes
1	cup chicken broth
1	clove garlic, minced
	1/2 tsp. each thyme and oregano
	Salt and pepper to taste

Shake chicken in plastic bag with flour; shake off excess and brown on both sides in large skillet with 1 Tbsp. olive oil. Add remaining ingredients and simmer until chicken is tender (about 45 minutes).

Yield: 4 servings   Count: 3 PRO 2 VEG

Crisp Crusted Fish

1	Tbsp. light ranch dressing
1	large egg white
3	Tbsp. yellow cornmeal
2	Tbsp. (1/2 ounce) fresh grated Parmesan cheese
2	Tbsp. flour
1/4	tsp. red ground pepper
1/8	tsp. salt
4	4 oz. pieces white fish

Combine dressing and egg white in small bowl. Combine remaining dry ingredients in plastic bag. Dip fish in egg mixture, then coat with dry ingredients in plastic bag. Place fish on baking sheet sprayed with nonstick spray. Bake at 425 degrees for 8 minutes; turn over and bake another 8 minutes or until lightly browned. Serve with lemon wedge.

Yield: 4 servings   Count: 3 PRO

Egg White Omelet

1/4	cup green onion
4	large egg whites
	Salt and white pepper to taste

In skillet coated with nonstick spray, sauté onion until soft. Set half aside. Beat egg whites until soft peaks form. Pour into pan and cook about 1 minute; top will turn white. Pull cooked part to center and cook remainder; add remaining onion; fold in half to complete cooking. Serve with chunky salsa.

Yield: 1 serving   Count: 2 PRO

Flank Steak

1	Tbsp. brown sugar
2	tsp. Kosher salt
1	tsp. cumin
1/2	tsp. five spice powder
1/4	tsp. ginger
1	lb. flank steak

Combine first 5 ingredients and sprinkle on steak. Grill for 6 minutes per side; cut steak across grain into thin slices.

Yield: 4 servings   Count: 3 PRO

Germaine's Chicken

6	4 oz. chicken breasts
1/2	cup hot water with 1 beef or chicken bouillon cube
1	pkg. frozen artichoke hearts, sliced
2-3	cloves garlic, sliced
1/4	tsp. rosemary
1/4	cup red wine

Combine all ingredients in baking pan, cover and bake for 30 minutes at 350 degrees. Remove cover and bake an additional 10 to 15 minutes.

Yield: 6 servings   Count: 3 PRO 1/2 VEG

Glazed Sesame Pork

4	4 oz. boneless center cut pork chops
1/4	tsp. each salt and pepper
3/4	cup chicken broth
2	Tbsp. sesame seeds, toasted
1	Tbsp. brown sugar
2	Tbsp. red wine vinegar
1	Tbsp. Dijon mustard

Brown chops on both sides in pan sprayed with nonstick spray. Add remaining ingredients, cover and simmer for 20 minutes. Uncover and simmer 20 minutes more or until tender.

Yield: 4 servings   Count: 3 PRO

Greek Scampi

1	tsp. olive oil
5	garlic cloves, minced
3	28 oz. can tomatoes, drained and chopped
1/2	cup fresh parsley, chopped
1-1/4	lb. large shrimp, peeled and de-veined
1	cup (4 oz.) feta cheese
2	Tbsp. lemon juice
1/4	tsp. pepper

Heat oil in large pan. Add garlic and sauté for 30 seconds. Add tomatoes and 1/2 parsley; reduce heat and simmer 10 minutes. Add shrimp and cook 5 minutes. Pour mixture into 13 by 9 baking dish; sprinkle with cheese and bake at 400 degrees for 10 minutes.

Sprinkle with remaining parsley, lemon juice, and pepper.

Yield: 6 servings   Count: 2 VEG 3 PRO

Herbed Chicken

1	tsp. oil
1-1/2	cups sliced mushrooms
1/2	cup onion, chopped
1	clove garlic, minced
1	lb. boneless, skinless chicken breast
1/2	tsp. each salt and basil
1/4	tsp. pepper
2	cups tomato, chopped

Sauté vegetables in oil for 2 minutes; add remaining ingredients; cover and simmer until chicken is done, about 20 minutes.

Yield: 4 servings   Count: 3 PRO 2 VEG

Lamb and Eggplant Loaf

1	medium eggplant
1	cup chopped onion
2	cloves garlic, minced
1/2	cup (2 oz.) feta cheese
1/3	cup uncooked bulgur
2	Tbsp. parsley, minced
2	Tbsp. lemon juice
2	tsp. fresh mint
1/4	tsp. each coriander, cumin, pepper
2	egg whites
1	lb. lean ground lamb

Pierce eggplant with fork and bake in 350 degree oven for 45 minutes. Cool, then peel and chop. Combine with remaining ingredients. Bake in loaf pan at 350 degrees for 1 hour and 10 minutes.

Yield: 6 servings   Count: 3 PRO 1/2 CHO

Lamb Vindaloo

1	lb. lamb sirloin, cut into 2" cubes
2	Tbsp. each coriander and turmeric
1	tsp. each cayenne and cumin
1/2	tsp. each fenugreek and black mustard
4	Tbsp. vinegar or lemon juice
1	medium onion, minced
4	cloves garlic, minced
1″	piece fresh ginger, grated

2	Tbsp. canola oil
1/2-3/4	cup tomato juice (to cover)
2	serrano peppers, finely minced
	Salt and pepper to taste

Mix the dry spices and vinegar to form a paste. Coat the lamb with the paste and then add onion, garlic, and ginger. Marinate at least 4 hours. Brown lamb in oil in small batches, seasoning with salt and pepper. When the lamb is browned, return it to the pot and add the tomato juice. Cover and simmer for about 1 hour until tender. Add the serranos.

Yield: 4 servings   Count: 3 PRO

Lemon Rosemary Chicken

2	medium lemons
1/2	tsp. dried rosemary
2	tsp. olive oil
1/2	tsp. salt
1/4	tsp. black pepper
1	clove garlic, minced
4	4 oz. skinless chicken breasts

Grate lemon to yield 2 tsp. peel. Slice one half of second lemon and save for garnish. Squeeze remaining lemons and combine with next five ingredients. Spray skillet with nonstick spray, and heat pan over medium heat. Toss chicken breasts in lemon mixture, then place in hot skillet. Cook 5 minutes a side, brushing with lemon mixture. Cook until juices are clear. Garnish with lemon slices.

Yield: 4 servings.   Count: 3 PRO

Lemongrass Roasted Chicken from Angie Eakin

1	Tbsp. lemongrass, finely chopped
3	Tbsp. cilantro stems and leaves
5	peppercorns
1	clove garlic, chopped
1	Tbsp. each canola oil, soy sauce, brown sugar and lime juice
1	tsp. each sea salt and chili flakes
1	lb. boneless, skinless chicken breasts

Using a food processor combine all ingredients except chicken and process until smooth. Pour into re-closeable plastic bag and add chicken. Marinate overnight. Grill, turning once until juices are clear. Baste with sauce while cooking. To serve, pour remaining sauce over chicken.

Sauce

1	Tbsp. canola oil
1	clove garlic, chopped
1/2	cup sugar
1/2	tsp. sea salt
2/3	cup apple cider vinegar
1/3	cup water
1	tsp. each red and cayenne pepper
2	Tbsp. each cilantro and lemongrass

Heat oil and add garlic; cook until golden; add remaining ingredients except cilantro and bring to boil. Reduce heat and simmer 15 minutes, until the sauce coats a spoon. Stir in cilantro just before serving.

Yield: 4 servings   Count: 3 PRO 1-1/2 CHO

Mexican Chicken Breasts

4   4 oz. chicken breasts, boneless and skinless
3   Tbsp. lime juice
1   tsp. each cumin, coriander, salt and sugar
1/8   tsp. pepper
1   Tbsp. chopped cilantro or parsley

Combine juice and seasonings; add to chicken; marinate for 30 min. Cook in pan sprayed with nonstick spray. Cook 5 to 6 minutes per side or until juices run clear. Brush with marinade half way through cooking. Garnish with cilantro.

Yield: 4 servings   Count: 3 PRO

Mexican Strata

1	cup salsa
1	cup canned black beans, rinsed and drained
5	corn tortillas, cut into strips
1	cup reduced fat cheese
1	cup low fat or tofu sour cream
1	cup nonfat or soy milk
1/2	tsp. salt
2	eggs plus 2 egg whites
1/4	cup green onion, sliced

Combine beans and salsa. Place 1/3 tortilla strips in 11 by 7 baking dish coated with nonstick spray. Top with 1/2 salsa mix and 1/3 cheese. Repeat, ending with remaining tortilla strips. Combine remaining ingredients and pour over all. Top with remaining 1/3 cheese. Cover with foil and chill overnight. Bake at 350 degrees for 20 minutes; remove cover and bake additional 10 minutes until lightly browned.

Yield: 6 servings.   Count: 2 PRO 1 CHO

Mustard Pork Tenderloin

1	lb. pork tenderloin
2	Tbsp. Dijon mustard
1	tsp. rosemary
1/2	tsp. salt
1/4	tsp. pepper

Preheat oven to 425 degrees. Spray baking pan with non-stick spray. Spread mustard on top of pork and sprinkle with seasonings. Bake for 30 minutes. To serve, slice into 1/4-inch slices and divide into four servings.

Yield: 4 servings   Count: 3 PRO

Orange Roughy with Tomato Coulis

2	cup tomato, chopped
1/4	tsp. salt
3	Tbsp. red wine vinegar
2	Tbsp. cilantro, chop
1	Tbsp. onion, minced
1	Tbsp. olive oil
1	clove garlic, crushed
1	lb. orange roughy
2	tsp. lemon rind
1/4	each tsp. salt and pepper

Drain chopped tomato in colander for 30 minutes. Add salt through garlic, stir well, and set aside. Sprinkle fish with lemon rind, salt and pepper. Broil or bake for 4 to 5 minutes per side. Serve with tomato coulis.

Yield: 4 servings   Count: 3 PRO 1 VEG

Oven Baked Chicken

1/4	cup breadcrumbs
1	Tbsp. Parmesan cheese
1	tsp. paprika
1	tsp. thyme
1/2	tsp. garlic salt
1/4	tsp. pepper
1/3	cup low fat buttermilk or soy milk
4	4 oz. chicken breasts, skinless and boneless

Combine dry ingredients in plastic bag. Dip chicken in milk and then shake in crumbs. Bake in nonstick pan at 400 degrees for 40 minutes.

Yield: 4 servings   Count: 3 PRO

Pasta Frittata

1/2	cup broken dry angel hair pasta
2	tsp. olive oil
1	small onion, sliced
1	red pepper, diced
6	large egg whites
2	large eggs
1/3	cup grated Parmesan or Pecorino Romano cheese
1/4	cup nonfat or soy milk
1/2	tsp. salt

Cook pasta until tender; drain. In non-stick, oven-proof pan, heat olive oil on stovetop. Add vegetables and stir fry until tender. In large bowl, combine remaining ingredients. Pour over vegetable mix and pasta. Cover and cook 3 minutes. Uncover and bake in 425 degree oven for 6 minutes or until set in center.

Yield: 4 servings   Count: 2 PRO 1/2 CHO

Pepper and Beef Stir Fry

1	lb. flank steak, thinly sliced across grain
1	cup pea pods
2	each red, yellow and green peppers
1	clove garlic, minced
4	green onions
2	tsp. cornstarch
1	pkt. Splenda or other sugar substitute
1/2	tsp. each ginger, salt and pepper
1	tsp. olive or canola oil
1/4	cup beef broth
2	Tbsp. soy sauce

Combine cornstarch thru soy sauce and set aside. Heat oil in large fry pan; add onion and garlic. Add beef slices and stir-fry until done; remove and set aside. Add vegetables and cook about 4 minutes until crisp-tender. Add beef mix back. Add sauce mix, stir, and cook until thickened.

Yield: 4 servings   Count: 3 PRO 2 VEG

Pizza Frittata

1/4	cup water
1/4	tsp. each salt and pepper
2	8 oz. carton egg substitute
2	4 oz. links sweet turkey sausage
1/2	cup onion, finely chopped
1	cup cherry tomato, halved
1	cup canned cannellini beans, rinsed and drained

Combine first four ingredients; set aside. Heat large non-stick skillet; add sausage and onion; cook 4 minutes; add tomatoes and cook 2 minutes, stirring frequently. Add beans. Pour egg mix over all, cover and cook for 3 minutes.

Yield: 4 servings   Count: 3 PRO 1 CHO

Pork Chops with Tomatoes

1	tsp. each cumin and chili powder
2	tsp. cider vinegar
1/2	tsp. cinnamon
4	4 oz. center-cut pork chops
1	tsp. oil
1	16 oz. pkg. frozen corn, thawed
1-1/2	cups red bell pepper, chopped
1/2	cup green onion, chopped
4	tsp. minced garlic
1	tsp. oregano
1	14.5 oz. can diced tomatoes, drained

Combine first four ingredients and coat both sides of chops. Heat oil in nonstick pan and brown chops on both sides, about 3 minutes. Add remaining ingredients. Cover, reducing heat, and simmer for 45 minutes.

Yield: 4 servings.   Count: 3 PRO 1 CHO 2 VEG

Pork and Green Bean Stir Fry

1   lb. pork tenderloin, sliced thin
1/4   cup each soy sauce and chicken broth
2   tsp. cornstarch
1   lb. green beans
2   tsp. vegetable oil
2   cloves garlic, minced
1/2   tsp. ginger

Combine soy sauce, cornstarch and pork in plastic bag. Steam green beans for 5 minutes. Heat oil and Sauté garlic. Add pork mix and cook for 2 to 3 minutes. Add green beans, broth and ginger and simmer for 2 minutes. May be served over rice if desired.

Yield: 4 servings   Count: 3 PRO 1 VEG

Portabello Chili from Dee Taylor

1   Tbsp. olive oil
2   cup onion, chopped
1   cup carrot, chopped
3   medium Portobello mushrooms, stemmed and chopped
1   14 oz. can diced tomatoes
1-1/2 cup vegetable broth
1   Tbsp. Worcestershire sauce
1   tsp. each chili powder and coriander
1   Tbsp. maple syrup
3   15 oz. cans beans, drained and rinsed

Cook onion, carrot, and mushroom in oil until softened. Add remaining ingredients and bring to boil; reduce heat and simmer until heated through.

Yield: 6 servings   Count: 2 PRO 2 CHO 1 VEG

Roast Pork

1/2   cup apricot preserves
1   tsp. each salt and oregano
3/4   tsp. garlic powder
1/2   tsp. black pepper
3   lb. pork loin

Preheat oven to 425 degrees. Place preserves in small pan and heat over medium for about 10 minutes or until melted. Keep warm.

Combine spices and rub evenly over pork. Place pork on rack coated with nonstick spray. Place rack in shallow pan and bake for 30 minutes. Brush 1/4 preserves over pork. Bake an additional 10 minutes or until meat thermometer reads 155 degrees. Let stand 10 minutes before slicing.

Yield: 14 servings   Count: 3 PRO 1/2 CHO

Salmon with Mustard Sauce

4	4 oz. salmon fillets
1	Tbsp. butter or margarine
3	Tbsp. green onion, sliced
2	Tbsp. dry white wine or chicken broth
3/4	cup chicken broth
1	Tbsp. Dijon mustard
3/4	tsp. cornstarch
1	tsp. tarragon

Sprinkle fish with salt and pepper. Melt half the butter in non-stick skillet and cook fish about 3-4 minutes per side until it flakes. Remove and set aside. Melt remaining butter and sauté onions, add wine. Combine remaining ingredients in small bowl. Add to onion mix and stir with whisk. Bring to boil, reduce heat and simmer until reduced to about 3/4 cup. Spoon sauce over fish to serve.

Yield: 4 servings   Count: 3 PRO

Salmon with Stir-Fry Vegetables

4	4 oz. salmon fillets
1	tsp. sesame or other oil
1	cup carrot, julienne cut
3/4	lb. asparagus, cut in 2″ slices
1	red bell pepper, sliced
1/4	tsp. salt
1/8	tsp. pepper
1	yellow crookneck squash, sliced
1-1/3	cups cooked brown rice

Grill salmon fillets, about 3-4 minutes per side or until fish flakes easily with a fork. Set aside and keep warm.

Heat oil in skillet to medium high. Add vegetables and sauté about 5 minutes or until crisp-tender. Stir in seasonings. Serve each fish fillet with 1/3 cup rice and 1/4 of the vegetable mix.

Yield: 4 servings   Count: 3 PRO 1 CHO 2 VEG

Sesame Chicken Nuggets

1	lb. boneless, skinless chicken breasts, cut into 2″ pieces
1/4	tsp. salt
1/8	tsp. pepper
2	egg whites
1/2	cup sesame seeds, toasted
1/2	cup dry bread crumbs

Combine sesame seeds and crumbs in plastic bag. Mix egg whites in bowl. Sprinkle chicken with salt and pepper. Dip chicken in egg white then seed/crumb mix. Place on baking sheet sprayed with nonstick spray. Bake at 350 degrees for 15 minutes. Serve with mustard.

Yield: 4 servings   Count: 3 PRO 1/2 CHO

Shrimp with Spinach

1	lb. large shrimp, no-tail, frozen and pre-cooked
4	garlic cloves, minced
2	Tbsp. olive oil
3	Tbsp. lemon juice
1/4	tsp. each salt and pepper
10	oz. fresh spinach, torn into pieces
1/3	cup white wine or chicken broth

Defrost and drain shrimp in colander. Heat oil in large skillet; add garlic and shrimp. Cook for about 5 minutes or until heated through. Add spinach and remaining ingredients; after bringing to boil cook about 1 minute.

Yield: 4 servings   Count: 3 PRO 1 VEG

Smothered Chicken

4	4 oz. boneless, skinless chicken breasts
1	cup plain nonfat yogurt
1/2	tsp. cinnamon
1/2	tsp. cumin
2	garlic cloves, minced
1	cup onion, sliced
1	bay leaf
1	15 oz. can stewed tomatoes
2	Tbsp. parsley, chopped

Combine yogurt and seasonings. Put chicken in re-sealable plastic bag and add yogurt mix; marinate overnight. Spray skillet with nonstick spray and heat to medium. Add chicken and brown on both sides. Add remaining marinade and ingredients. Cover and simmer about 30 minutes or until chicken is tender.

Yield: 4 servings   Count: 3 PRO 1/2 VEG

Sole with Stewed Tomato

1/2	cup chopped onion
6	sole fillets, about 5 oz. each
1/2	cup dry white wine
1/2	cup diced, peeled, seeded tomato
1	tsp. salt
2	Tbsp. olive oil

Preheat oven to 400 degrees. Rinse onion in sieve for milder flavor. Arrange fish in a single layer in oven-proof pan; sprinkle with onion. Add the wine, tomato, and salt. Place a piece of aluminum foil on top and bake in center of oven for 10 to 12 minutes, until fish is cooked through. Remove fish. Bring juices to boil and reduce to about 2/3 cup. Add the oil and bring back to a boil; pour over fish to serve.

Yield: 6 servings   Count: 3 PRO

Spicy Chicken from Jana Stein

8	4 oz. boneless, skinless chicken breasts
2	Tbsp. lemon juice
2	Tbsp. olive or canola oil
4	cloves garlic
1	Tbsp. Kosher salt
3	Tbsp. brown sugar
1	tsp. oregano
1	Tbsp. red chili powder
1/4	cup cilantro, minced

Combine garlic through cilantro in food processor and blend into a paste. Place chicken in plastic re-sealable bag; combine lemon juice and oil and pour over chicken; add spicy paste and mix to coat chicken. Seal bag and place in refrigerator for 1 hour or longer. Pre-heat grill. Remove chicken pieces from marinade and grill 3 to 4 minutes per side, turning twice until juices run clear.

Yield: 8 servings   Count: 3 PRO

Spinach Salad with Sesame Pork

1	lb. pork tenderloin, sliced
2	Tbsp. soy sauce
1	Tbsp. honey
1/2	tsp. each ginger, pepper and garlic powder
1	Tbsp. each oil, rice vinegar and water
1/4	cup green onion, sliced
8	cups spinach leaves
4	tsp. sesame seeds

Combine soy sauce through garlic and coat pork; broil 4 minutes per side until juices are clear. Combine oil, vinegar and water and toss with spinach. Divide onto four plates; sprinkle with onion. Top with pork divided evenly; sprinkle with sesame seeds.

Yield: 4 servings   Count: 3 PRO 2 VEG

Spinach and Onion Frittata

6	large egg whites and 1 large egg yolk or 1 cup egg substitute
1	cup sweet onion, thinly sliced
2	Tbsp. water
1/4	tsp. sugar
1/8	tsp. pepper and nutmeg
4	cups spinach, torn

Preheat oven to 450 degrees. Cook onion slices in nonstick pan coated with spray until crisp tender. Add water and sugar and cook 5 minutes until tender and brown. Add spinach, cover and cook for 2 minutes. Add egg, pepper, and nutmeg. Bake for 5 to 10 minutes or until set.

Yield: 2 servings.   Count: 3 PRO 2 VEG

Sweet and Sour Chicken from Jana Stein

4   boneless, skinless chicken breasts
4   stalk celery, diced
2   red peppers, thinly sliced
1   8 oz. can pineapple chunks in juice
1/4   tsp. ground ginger
2   Tbsp. brown sugar
3   Tbsp. water
1-1/2   Tbsp. soy sauce
1   Tbsp. cider vinegar
1   Tbsp. cornstarch

Place chicken in microwave-safe dish. Sprinkle with salt and pepper and ginger; top with celery. Cover with waxed paper and microwave for 16 minutes. Drain pineapple; combine juice with remaining ingredients; microwave for 3 minutes, stirring once. Pour mixture over chicken, top with pineapple and pepper. Cook in microwave for 6 to 8 minutes.

Yield: 4 servings   Count: 3 PRO 1 CHO 1 VEG

Texas Turkey Patties

1	lb. ground turkey breast
2	green onion, chopped
1	zucchini, grated
1	carrot, grated
2	tsp. chili powder
3/4	tsp. salt
1/4	tsp. cumin
1/8	tsp. pepper

Combine all ingredients and shape into four patties. Spray pan with nonstick spray. Cook patties about 5 minutes per side or until juices run clear.

Yield: 4 servings   Count: 3 PRO 1/2 VEG

Turkey Burgers

1	lb. ground turkey
1/4	cup fresh parsley, minced
2	scallions, chopped
1/2	tsp. salt
1/4	tsp. black pepper
1/4	cup mango chutney, chopped

Combine all ingredients. Form into four patties. Grill or cook in nonstick pan coated with nonstick spray for 5 minutes per side or until juices are clear.

Yield: 4 servings   Count: 3 PRO

Turkey Chili

1	cup onion, diced
1	lb. turkey sausage, sliced
2	cups water
1	28 oz. can stewed tomatoes
1	tsp. each cumin, oregano, and chili powder
1/2	cup each celery and carrot, diced
1	clove garlic, minced
1/4	tsp. each salt and pepper
1	4 oz. can green chilies, chopped

Combine all ingredients in large pot and bring to a boil. Reduce heat and simmer for 30 minutes.

Yield: 4 servings   Count: 3 PRO 2 VEG

Turkey Meatloaf from Jane Taylor

1	cup chopped onion
3	cloves garlic, minced
1-1/4	lb. ground turkey
1/3	cup rolled oats
1	egg
1/2	cup tomato sauce
1	tsp. Worcestershire sauce
1/2	tsp. each salt and pepper

Mix all ingredients lightly and bake in loaf pan at 350 degrees for 1 hour.

Yield: 6 servings   Count: 3 PRO

Turkey Spinach Meatloaf

1-1/4 lb. ground turkey
1/2 box frozen chopped spinach, thawed and squeezed dry
2/3 cup instant mashed potatoes
1/2 cup shredded carrot
1/2 cup onion, chopped
1/4 cup marinara sauce
1 tsp. each garlic salt and Italian seasoning
1/4 tsp. pepper
1 egg

Mix all ingredients in medium bowl. Shape mixture into loaf and place on a shallow pan, that has been sprayed with nonstick spray. Bake for 50 to 60 minutes at 350 degrees.

Yield: 5 servings

Count: 3 PRO 1 VEG 1/2 CHO

Turkey Tortilla Casserole

1 cup onion, chopped
2 cloves garlic, minced
1 bunch Swiss chard, chopped
8 oz. sliced mushrooms
3/4 lb. ground turkey
4 corn tortilla, quartered
4 oz. grated reduced fat cheese
1 14 oz. can crushed tomatoes

Cook turkey in microwave proof dish for 3 minutes; stir and cook another 3 minutes; drain and set aside. Combine onion, garlic, chard and mushrooms; cover with plastic wrap and microwave for 2 to 3 minutes or until soft. In 11 by 8 inch pan sprayed with nonstick spray, spread vegetable mix and top with ground turkey. Pour crushed tomatoes over. Top with tortilla pieces and cheese. Bake at 375 degrees for 20 minutes.

Yield: 4 servings   Count: 3 PRO 2 VEG 1 CHO

Zucchini Frittata

2   cup thinly sliced zucchini
6   large eggs
1/2   cup low-fat grated cheese
2   Tbsp. parsley
         Garlic and onion to taste

Spray nonstick skillet. Combine all ingredients and cook until bottom is set. Cover to cook top.

Yield: 4 servings   Count: 2 PRO 1 VEG

Salads and Dressings

Asian Salad

6	chicken breasts, boneless and skinless
1/2	cup chicken broth
1	head iceberg lettuce, shredded
4	green onions, sliced
1/4	cup cilantro, chopped
1	4 oz. can water chestnuts, thinly sliced
3	stalks celery, thinly sliced
6	radishes, thinly sliced
2	Tbsp. sesame seeds, toasted
	Rice vinegar for dressing

Simmer chicken breasts in broth for 15 minutes or until done; remove from broth, cool, then chop. Combine remaining ingredients and divide into six servings.

Yield: 6 servings   Count: 3 PRO 2 VEG

Beet Salad

1	cup canned beets, chopped
1/2	cup frozen green peas, thawed
2	Tbsp. green onions, sliced
1	Tbsp. parsley, chopped
2	Tbsp. fat-free Italian dressing
	Lettuce leaves

Combine first four ingredients with dressing in bowl; cover and chill for 2 hours. Serve on lettuce leaves.

Yield: 4 servings   Count: 1 VEG

Bob's Broccoli Salad

4-1/2 cups broccoli florets
1/2   cup shredded soy cheese
1/2   cup soynuts
1/4   cup raisins
1   cup fat-free Miracle Whip
2   Tbsp. vinegar
1/2   cup Bacos
Combine all ingredients and chill.

Yield: 6 servings   Count: 1 CHO 1-1/2 PRO 1/2 VEG

Broccoli and Bean Salad

1-1/2 cups broccoli florets, chopped
2   Tbsp. red wine vinegar
2   tsp. olive or canola oil
1/4   tsp. pepper
1/8   tsp. salt
1   clove garlic, minced
1/4   cup each red bell pepper and red onion,
       chopped
1-1/2 cups white beans, rinsed
Steam broccoli until crisp tender. Add pepper, onion and beans. Combine remaining ingredients and stir well.

Yield: 4 servings   Count: 1/2 PRO 1/2 VEG 1 CHO

Carrot Salad

5   cups, sliced carrots
2   garlic cloves, halved
2/3   cup fresh lemon juice
1/4   cup chopped parsley
1   Tbsp. sugar
2
1   tsp. cinnamon

1/2   tsp. each cumin and paprika
Combine carrot and garlic in pan; cover with water. Cook about 8 minutes or until tender. Discard garlic. Combine remaining ingredients and stir to coat. Chill.

Makes 8 servings   Count: 1 VEG

Carrot Slaw

2   cups carrot, grated
1/3   cup dried cranberries
2   oz. walnut, chopped
3   Tbsp. mayonnaise
1/2 - 1   Tbsp. lemon juice
Combine all ingredients; chill.

Yield: 4 servings   Count: 1 VEG 1/2 CHO

Cauliflower Salad

2-1/2 cups cauliflower florets
2   Tbsp. parsley, chopped
2-1/2 Tbsp. lemon juice
1   tsp. olive oil
1/8   tsp. garlic powder
1/3   cup sliced radishes

Steam cauliflower 1 to 5 minutes or until crisp-tender. Rinse in cold water and drain. Combine next four ingredients and add to cauliflower and radishes.

Yield: 2 servings   Count: 1 VEG

Chicken and Asparagus Salad

2	cup asparagus, sliced
2	tsp. Dijon mustard
1	lb. boneless and skinless chicken breasts
1/4	tsp. salt
1/8	tsp. pepper
1	tsp. olive oil
1/3	cup green onion
4	cups salad greens

Steam asparagus until crisp tender. Coat chicken with mustard, salt and pepper; slice thinly. Heat oil and stir fry chicken and green onion. Cook until done and juices are clear. Add mix of 3 Tbsp. water, 2 Tbsp. white vinegar, 1 Tbsp. olive oil, 1 tsp. Dijon mustard and cook 1 minute. To serve, put 1 cup greens on salad plate; top with 1/2 cup asparagus and 1/4 chicken mix.

Yield: 4 servings   Count: 3 PRO 2 VEG

Chicken Salad

4	4 oz. chicken breast, no bone or skin, pounded thin
1	Tbsp. honey
1/3	cup cornflake crumbs
2	Tbsp. chopped pistachios
1	tsp. lemon rind
8	cups fancy salad greens
2	Tbsp. lemon juice

1   tsp. Dijon mustard

1   pkt. sugar substitute

1   tsp. olive oil

Brush chicken with honey. Combine crumbs, nuts, and rind in plastic bag; add chicken and shake to coat. Brown in nonstick pan adding salt and pepper to taste and cook about 5 minutes per side. Slice into strips. Combine lemon juice through oil, adding salt and pepper to taste. Add to salad greens and toss to coat. To serve, place 2 cups greens on plate and add 1 chicken breast, sliced.

Yield: 4 servings   Count: 3 PRO 2 VEG

Chicken Potato Salad

3/4   lb. red potato, quartered

2   tsp. olive oil

12   oz. cooked chicken breasts, cubed

1/4   cup green onion, chopped

1/4   cup white wine or chicken broth

1/4   cup white vinegar

2   Tbsp. fresh tarragon, chopped

2   Tbsp. fat-free mayonnaise

1   tsp. Dijon mustard

       Salt and pepper to taste

Place potato and oil in plastic bag; shake to coat. Bake in oven at 400 degrees for 20 minutes or until tender. Cool. Add chicken to potatoes and onion. Combine remaining ingredients and pour over chicken mix, stirring to coat.

Yield: 4 servings   Count: 3 PRO 1 CHO

Chicken Spinach Salad

1	bag pre-washed baby spinach
1	lb. asparagus, cut in 1-1/2″ pieces, steamed
1	red onion, sliced and steamed
1	lb. chicken tenders
1/2	tsp. salt
1/4	tsp. pepper
1	Tbsp. olive oil
1	Tbsp. balsamic vinegar
1	Tbsp. lemon juice
1/2	tsp. Dijon mustard
1/4	tsp. sugar

Place spinach on four plates. Steam asparagus and onion; divide and place on top of spinach. Stir-fry chicken in pan coated with nonstick spray; cook until done and juices are clear; divide and add on top vegetable mix. Combine remaining ingredients and drizzle over salad.

Yield: 4 servings   Count: 3 PRO 3 VEG

Chicken and Strawberry Spinach Salad

4	4 oz. boneless, skinless chicken breasts
8	cups baby spinach leaves
1	cup strawberries, hulled and cut in half

Dressing: combine 3 Tbsp. apple juice, 2 Tbsp. strawberry spreadable fruit and 2 Tbsp. balsamic vinegar.

Grill or cook chicken breasts as desired; season to taste. Divide spinach onto four serving plates. Slice chicken and arrange on top of greens. Add strawberries; drizzle with dressing.

Yield: 4 servings   Count: 3 PRO 2 VEG 1/2 CHO

Chinese Chicken Salad

6   4 oz. chicken breasts, boneless and skinless
1/2   cup chicken broth
1   head iceberg lettuce, shredded
4   green onions, sliced
1/4   cup cilantro, chopped
1   4 oz. can water chestnuts, thinly sliced
3   stalks celery
6   radishes, thinly sliced
2   Tbsp. sesame seeds, toasted
       Rice vinegar for dressing

Simmer chicken breasts in broth for 15 minutes or until done. Remove from broth, cool, then chop. Combine with remaining ingredients and divide onto serving plates.

Yield: 6 servings.   Count: 3 PRO 2 VEG

Copper Penny Salad

2	cups carrots, sliced and cooked
1	medium onion, sliced thinly
1	medium green pepper, sliced thinly
1/3	cup vinegar
2	Tbsp. oil
1/2	tsp. dry mustard
6	pkt. sugar substitute
1/2	tsp. Worcestershire
1/4	tsp. salt
1/2	can condensed tomato soup

Mix vinegar through soup and combine with vegetables; marinate overnight.

Yield: 8 servings   Count: 1 VEG

Green Bean Salad

1	lb. fresh green beans
12	cherry tomato, halved
1/4	cup chopped red onion
1/3	cup chopped fresh parsley
2	Tbsp. each water and white vinegar
2	Tbsp. parmesan cheese (use sheep cheese for milk-free)
1	Tbsp. olive oil
1/4	tsp. thyme and pepper
1	clove garlic, minced.

Steam beans until crisp tender. Chill. Combine with tomato and onion. Combine remaining ingredients and toss to coat.

Yield: 6 servings   Count: 2 VEG

Low-Carb Potato Salad

1-1/2 head cauliflower
4   small potatoes, steamed and cubed
¼   cup instant mashed potato granules
½   cup mayonnaise
2   tsp. mustard
1/2   cup dill pickle, chopped
5   hard cooked eggs, diced
1/4   cup olives, sliced
        Salt, pepper, herbs to taste

Steam cauliflower florets until crisp-tender. Combine remaining ingredients and chill.

Yield: 14 servings   Count: 1/2 CHO 1 FAT

Oriental Beef Salad

1	lb. beef top round steak
1/3	cup orange juice
1/4	cup low sodium soy sauce
2	Tbsp. rice vinegar
1	tsp. each cornstarch and oil
1/2	tsp. ground ginger
1/4	tsp. pepper
8	oz. shredded cabbage
5	oz. shredded carrot (1-1/2 cup)
3	green onion, chopped
4	leaves butter lettuce

Trim all fat from beef and cut in half, then in 1/8″ slices. Heat oil in pan and stir-fry beef until just done. Remove and set aside. Combine remaining ingredients, excluding lettuce and stir-fry about 1 minute; add beef and heat. Serve on lettuce leaves.

Yield: 4 servings   Count: 3 PRO 1 VEG

Persimmon Salad

1	box sugar-free orange gelatin
2	cups hot water
2	Tbsp. lemon juice
1-1/2	cups cold water
1	cup persimmon pulp (about 2)
1/4	cup pecans, toasted and chopped
1	orange, peeled and sectioned

Dissolve gelatin in hot water. Add lemon juice and cold water. When chilled and syrupy, add remaining ingredients. Chill until set. Serve on leaf lettuce.

Yield: 8 servings   Count: 1/2 CHO

Pineapple Salad

1   20 oz. can crushed pineapple in juice
1   large box orange sugar-free gelatin
2   cup buttermilk
8   oz. light Cool Whip

Bring pineapple to boil; add gelatin and stir until dissolved. Add buttermilk and cool to room temperature. Fold in whipped topping. Pour into pan or mold and refrigerate overnight.

Yield: 10 servings   Count: 1 CHO

Pork Tenderloin Salad

1	1 lb. pork tenderloin
2	Tbsp. dry sherry
4-1/2	tsp. soy sauce
1/4	tsp. ginger
8	cups leaf lettuce
1	10 oz. pkg. frozen peas, thawed
2	Tbsp. fat free mayonnaise
2	Tbsp. balsamic vinegar
1	Tbsp. Dijon mustard
1	tsp. sugar
1/4	tsp. pepper

Cut pork into thin slices; combine with sherry, soy, and ginger. Spray nonstick pan with nonstick spray. Cook over medium high heat, stirring constantly until pork loses its pink color. Combine last five ingredients and toss with lettuce. Divide onto four serving dishes and top with pork and peas.

Yield: 4 servings   Count: 3 PRO 1 CHO 2 VEG

Salmon and Potato Salad

2	Tbsp. water
2	Tbsp. lemon juice
1/2	tsp. lemon rind
2	Tbsp. fat free mayonnaise
1/8	tsp. each salt and pepper
1	lb. salmon fillet

8   small red potatoes, quartered
2   1/2″ slices onion
1/2   tsp. dill
1/3   cup celery, diced

Combine first 5 ingredients and set aside. Place salmon, potatoes, onion in steamer; sprinkle with dill. Steam for 15 minutes. Flake fish and combine with mayo mix and celery.

Yield: 4 servings   Count: 3 PRO 1 CHO

Sesame Chicken Salad

2   cups cooked chicken breast
2   cups Napa cabbage, thinly sliced
1   cup red bell pepper strips
1   cup each fresh bean sprouts and grated carrot
2   Tbsp. green onion, chopped
1   tsp. sesame seed, toasted

Combine all ingredients in large bowl. Top with dressing and sesame seeds.

Dressing: combine 1/4 cup each rice vinegar and reduced sodium soy sauce, 2 Tbsp. creamy peanut butter, 1 tsp each vegetable oil and minced garlic, 1/4 tsp. Ginger.

Yield: 4 servings   Count: 3 PRO 2 VEG

Shrimp Salad

2	Tbsp. olive oil
2	Tbsp. white vinegar
1	Tbsp. lemon juice
1/2	tsp. dill
1/8	tsp. dry mustard
1	clove garlic, crushed
3/4	cup low fat jack cheese, cubed
1	lb. cooked baby shrimp
1	cucumber, sliced
	Romaine lettuce

Combine first six ingredients. Mix with shrimp and cheese. Serve on romaine with cucumber slices.

Yield: 8 servings   Count: 3 PRO

Shrimp and Tomato Salad

12	cups gourmet salad greens
1/2	cup red onion, chopped
2	each green, yellow and red tomato, sliced
1-1/8	lb. frozen pre-cooked shrimp
	Tony Baloney's Rossa Fat Free Italian dressing

Defrost shrimp and drain on paper towels. Divide greens onto six plates; top with red onion. Divide tomato slices and arrange around edge of plate. Divide shrimp evenly to top of each salad.

Yield: 6 servings   Count: 3 VEG 3 PRO 1 CHO

Smoked Chicken and Potato Salad

4   small red potatoes, diced and steamed

1   12 oz. package smoked chicken sausage, quartered and sliced

1   cup celery, chopped

1/2   cup each carrot and red onion, chopped

1/4   cup Dijon mustard

2   Tbsp. lemon juice

      Salt and pepper to taste

Combine all ingredients and toss to coat.

Yield: 4 servings   Count: 3 PRO 1 CHO 1 VEG

Spinach Salad with Oranges

1/4   cup chopped nuts

1   Tbsp. orange juice

1   Tbsp. olive or canola oil

1   tsp. Dijon mustard

1/4   tsp. each salt and pepper

1   7 oz. pkg. fresh baby spinach

2   oranges, peeled and sectioned

Place nuts in microwave and cook for 45-60 seconds or until toasted. Set aside. Combine next four ingredients and pour over spinach; mix to coat. Divide spinach on salad plates; top with orange sections and nuts.

Yield: 4 servings   Count: 2 VEG 1/2 CHO

Spinach Mushroom Salad

1	10 oz. bag fresh spinach
1	8 oz. pkg. sliced mushrooms
1/2	cup red onion rings (optional)
2	Tbsp. sesame seed
3	Tbsp. cider vinegar
2	Tbsp. each water and honey
1	Tbsp. Dijon mustard
1	Tbsp. canola or olive oil
1/2	tsp. pepper
1	garlic clove, minced

Tear spinach into bite size pieces and combine with mushrooms and onion. Combine remaining ingredients in jar and shake well. Pour over salad and toss.

Yield: 5 servings   Count: 2 VEG 1 FAT

Spinach Cauliflower Salad

2	cups spinach leaves, torn
1	cup leaf lettuce, torn
1	cup cauliflower florets
1	cup mushrooms, sliced
1/2	cup yellow bell pepper, sliced
1/2	cup red onion, sliced
2	Tbsp. lemon juice
1-1/2	tsp. sugar
1/2	tsp. thyme
2	tsp. water

1-1/2 tsp. olive oil

1/4   tsp. black pepper

Combine first six ingredients in large bowl; combine remaining ingredients and pour over spinach mix; toss gently to coat.

Yield: 4 servings   Count: 1 VEG

Sweet Coleslaw

3   cup shredded cabbage

1   cup shredded carrot

3   oz. dried cranberries

1   cup rice vinegar

4 to 6 pkt. sugar substitute

1   tsp. each celery and mustard seed

Combine all ingredients and chill; divide into six servings.

Yield: 6 servings   Count: 1/2 CHO 1 VEG

Taco Salad

3/4	lb. ground round or turkey
2	cup chopped red or yellow bell pepper
2	cups salsa
1	bag salad greens (dark green is best)
2	small tomato, chopped
4	oz. shredded low-fat cheese
4	oz. baked tortilla chips
1/4	cup green onion, chopped

Cook meat and bell pepper until meat is browned; stir to crumble; pour off any liquid. Add salsa and bring to boil. Divide greens evenly among four plates; top each with 1/4th meat mixture; divide remaining ingredients onto each plate.

Yield: 4 servings   Count: 3 PRO 2 VEG 1 CHO

Three Bean Salad

1	16 oz. can canned kidney beans, drained and rinsed
1	8 oz. can each green beans, yellow wax beans, and sliced carrots, drained and rinsed
1	bell pepper, chopped
1/2	cup red onion, chopped
1/4	cup cider vinegar
3	pkt. Splenda or other sugar substitute
2	tsp. Dijon mustard
1	clove garlic, minced

1   tsp. basil
2   Tbsp. canola or olive oil

Combine beans, carrots, pepper and onion in large bowl. In a small bowl combine remaining ingredients. Pour over bean mixture and stir. Chill.

Yield: 8 servings   Count: 1/2 CHO 1 VEG

Tomato and Cucumber Salad with Feta

2   cups diced tomato (about 1 lb.)
1   cup diced English cucumber
1/4   cup (1 oz.) crumbled feta cheese (sheep or goat if desired)
1   Tbsp. finely chopped fresh mint

Combine all ingredients and combine with vinaigrette dressing of choice.

Yield: 4 servings   Count: 1 VEG

Waldorf Salad

3	medium apples, peeled and diced
2	tsp. lemon juice
1-1/2	cups seedless grapes, halved
1	cup celery, diced
1/3	cup raisins
1/4	cup walnuts, toasted, chopped
1/4	cup reduced calorie mayonnaise
1/4	cup nonfat buttermilk
1	pkt. Splenda or other sugar substitute

Combine apples and lemon juice; add grapes, celery, raisin and walnuts. Combine remaining ingredients and stir into apple mix. Refrigerate 1 hour.

Yield: 8 servings   Count: 1 CHO

White Bean and Chicken Salad

2	cups chicken, cooked and diced
1	cup tomato, chopped
1/2	cup red onion, chopped
1/4	cup fresh basil, chopped
1	16 oz. can cannellini beans, rinsed and drained
1/4	cup red wine vinegar
2	Tbsp. olive oil
1	Tbsp. fresh lemon juice
2	tsp. mustard
1/2	tsp. salt
1/4	tsp. pepper

2   garlic cloves, minced

Combine first five ingredients; then combine remaining ingredients and toss gently.

Yield: 4 servings   Count: 4 PRO 1 CHO 1 VEG

Balsamic Vinaigrette

1   cup low sodium chicken broth
2   tsp. cornstarch or arrowroot
1   clove garlic clove, minced
1/4   cup white wine vinegar
3   Tbsp. balsamic vinegar
1   tsp. Dijon mustard
1/2   tsp. dried basil

Combine broth, cornstarch, and garlic in saucepan. Boil for 1 minute, stirring constantly. Remove from heat and add remaining ingredients. Cover and chill.

Yield: 12 servings   Count: FREE

Dijon Vinaigrette

1/2	cup chicken broth
1/2	cup balsamic vinegar
2	Tbsp. olive oil
2	tsp. Dijon mustard
1/4	tsp. black pepper
3	cloves garlic, minced

Combine all ingredients in jar and shake to combine. Chill 1 hour. Drizzle over salad greens.

Yield: 1-1/4 cup   Count: 2 Tbsp. = FREE
                                    4 Tbsp. = 1 FAT

Garlic Dressing

1-2	cloves garlic, crushed
1/4	lb. firm tofu
1/4	cup water
3	Tbsp. lemon juice
1	Tbsp. soy sauce
1	Tbsp. tahini
1	Tbsp. chopped fresh dill
1	tsp. honey
	Pepper to taste

Blend all ingredients until smooth and creamy; chill before serving.

Yield: 6 servings   Count: FREE

Poppy Seed Dressing

1	12.3 oz. box reduced fat tofu
1/4	cup Mocha Mix Fat-Free
1	tsp. Dijon mustard
2	tsp. apple cider vinegar
2	Tbsp. catsup
2	tsp. grated onion
1/3	tsp. dry mustard
1	Tbsp. lemon juice
1	tsp. poppy seeds

Blend all ingredients until smooth.

Yield: 10 servings   Count: FREE

Tofu Caesar Dressing

1	12.3 oz. box soft light tofu
1/4	cup olive oil
1/4	cup water
1/4	cup lemon juice
1	Tbsp. anchovy paste (optional)
2	Tbsp. red wine vinegar
2	Tbsp. Parmesan cheese (goat or sheep for milk-free)
1	Tbsp. Dijon mustard
1	clove garlic, minced
1/2	tsp. pepper

Blend all ingredients until smooth; store tight fitting container.

Yield: 16 servings   Count = 1 FAT

Tofu Pesto

1-1/2 cups fresh basil
1/2   cup Mori Nu Silken tofu
1/4   cup pine nuts
1   Tbsp. olive oil
1   clove garlic
       Salt and pepper to taste
Blend all ingredients in food processor until smooth.

Yield: 6 servings   Count: 1 PRO

Spicy Tomato Dressing

1   5.5 oz. can spicy hot vegetable juice
3   Tbsp. red wine vinegar
1   Tbsp. olive oil
1   clove garlic, crushed
1/2   tsp. sugar
1/2   tsp. dry mustard
Combine all ingredients in container and shake to blend.
Refrigerate; shake before using.

Yield: 8 servings   Count: FREE

Vinaigrette Dressing

1	cup vegetable broth
2	tsp. cornstarch
2	Tbsp. red wine vinegar
1	Tbsp. olive oil
1	tsp. sugar
1/4	tsp. salt
1/8	tsp. black pepper

Combine broth and cornstarch in saucepan, stirring with whisk. Bring to boil over medium heat; cook 1 minute, stirring constantly. Remove from heat and stir in remaining ingredients. Cover and chill. Stir before using.

Yield: 16 servings   Count: FREE

Variations:

—add 2 tsp. Dijon mustard
—add 2 tsp. bottled minced roasted garlic
—omit vinegar and add 3 Tbsp. fresh lime juice and 1/4 tsp. cumin

Breads

Blueberry French Toast

12	slices day-old bread, crusts removed and cubed
2	8 oz. pkg. light cream cheese, cubed
1	cup fresh or frozen blueberries
24	oz. egg substitute (equal to 12 eggs)
2	cups skim milk and 1/3 cup maple syrup

Coat 13 by 9 by 2 inch pan with nonstick spray. Place half of bread cubes in pan. Top with cheese cubes, then add blueberries and remaining bread. Combine egg substitute, milk and syrup and pour over bread mixture. Cover and chill 8 hours or overnight. Remove from refrigerator 30 minutes before baking. Bake at 350 degrees for 30 minutes. Uncover and bake 30 minutes or until set.

Yield: 12 servings   Count: 1 CHO 1-1/2 PRO

Carrot Sweet Potato Muffins

2-3/4	cup flour
1/2	cup each white and brown sugar
1	Tbsp. baking powder
1	tsp. each baking soda, salt, cinnamon
1/2	tsp. allspice
1-1/4	cup grated carrot
1-1/4	cup milk (non-dairy substitute if desired)
1/3	box (4.1 oz.) reduced fat tofu

1/2	cup mashed sweet potato or pumpkin
1/4	cup oil
1	Tbsp. vanilla
1	egg white plus 1 egg

Combine flour through allspice; stir in carrot. Combine milk and remaining ingredients. Add to flour mix, stirring just until moist. Spoon batter into muffin cups coated with nonstick spray. Bake at 400 degrees for 10 to 15 minutes. Remove immediately and cool on wire rack.

Yield: 24   Count: 1 CHO

Cheese Biscotti

2-3/4   cup flour
3/4   cup sharp cheddar cheese (may use goat cheddar)
1/2   cup fresh Parmesan cheese (may use Pecorino Romano)
2   tsp. baking powder
3/4   tsp. salt
1/4   cup nonfat milk (may use soy)
2   tsp. canola oil
3   large eggs

Preheat oven to 350 degrees. Combine flour through salt. Combine milk, oil and eggs; add to flour mix and stir until well-blended (mixture will be dry and crumbly). Turn onto floured board and knead 10 times. Divide dough in half. Shape each into a roll. Place on baking sheet sprayed with nonstick spray. Flatten to 1″ thickness. Bake at 350 degrees for 30 minutes. Remove from baking sheet; cool on wire rack for 10 minutes. Reduce oven to 325 degrees. Cut each roll into 10 slices; place cut side down and bake for 10 minutes; turn over and repeat. Cool on wire rack.

Yield: 20   Count: 1 CHO 1/2 PRO

Cheese Biscuits

3   whole eggs, slightly beaten
1-1/2   cups soy flour
2   Tbsp. baking powder
2   Tbsp. oil

1/2   cup sour cream
1/4   cup water—add slowly
1-1/2 cups grated cheddar cheese
1/4   tsp. salt

Combine dry ingredients in mixing bowl. In separate bowl combine eggs, oil, and sour cream; add to dry ingredients; add water and mix gently (do not over mix). Drop by tablespoons onto large greased cookie sheet, making four rows of four each. Bake 12 to 15 minutes or until golden brown. Cool for 10 minutes. Refrigerate or freeze.

Yield: 16   Count: 1/3 CHO 1 PRO

Pumpkin or Persimmon Bread

1-1/2 cups Splenda
1/4   tsp. baking powder
1   tsp. baking soda
3/4   tsp. salt
1/2   tsp. each cloves, nutmeg, cinnamon, ginger
1-2/3 cup flour
1/2   cup each oil and water
1   cup pumpkin or persimmon pulp
1/2   cup egg substitute
1/2   cup chopped pecans
1/4   cup raisins

Mix dry ingredients, add remaining ingredients. Bake in loaf pan sprayed with nonstick spray at 325 to 350 degrees for 1 hr.

Yield: 16 servings   Count: 1 CHO

Strawberry Orange Muffins

1-1/4	cup strawberries, sliced
2	Tbsp. margarine, melted
2	tsp. orange rind
2	large eggs
1-1/2	cup flour
1	cup sugar
1	tsp. baking powder
1/2	tsp. salt

Preheat oven to 400 degrees; spray muffin tin cups with nonstick spray. Blend berries, margarine, rind and eggs together. Combine flour, sugar, baking powder and salt. Add berry mixture and stir just until moist. Spoon batter into cups and sprinkle with sugar. Bake for 20 min. Remove from pan immediately and cool on rack.

Yield: 12 muffins   Count: 2 CHO

Wheat Bran Muffins

1/2	cup brown sugar
1/4	cup shortening
1/2	cup Splenda
2	eggs
1	cup soy milk
1-1/2	cups bran
1/2	cup each white and whole wheat flours
1-1/2	tsp. baking soda
	Pinch salt

1/4   cup raisins

1/2   cup soynuts

Mix first five ingredients with electric mixer; combine bran through salt; add and mix quickly. Fold in raisins and nuts. Spoon into muffin tins which have been sprayed with non-stick spray and bake at 400 degrees for 12 to 15 minutes or until done.

Yield: 18   Count:1 CHO

Desserts

Almond Meringue Cookies

4	egg whites
1	tsp. cream of tartar
1/4	tsp. salt
1	cup sugar
1	tsp. each grated orange peel and vanilla
1/4	tsp. almond extract
1	cup sliced almonds

Beat egg whites with cream of tartar and salt until frothy. Beating on high, gradually add in sugar, beating until stiff peaks form. Fold in remaining ingredients. Drop teaspoons onto cookie sheet coated with nonstick spray. Bake 300 degrees for 15 to 20 minutes.

Yield: 4 dozen.   Count: 3 cookies = 1 CHO

Almond Pumpkin Pie

16	Amaretti cookies, crushed
1	egg white
2	cups canned pumpkin
1-1/3	cup low-fat or soy milk
1/2	cup brown sugar
1	Tbsp. flour
3	Tbsp. Amaretto
1/2	tsp. salt
1-1/2	tsp. each cinnamon and vanilla

1/4 tsp. each ginger and almond extract

2 egg whites

1 egg

Combine cookie crumbs and egg white; press into 9″ pan sprayed with nonstick spray. Bake at 375 degrees for 10 minutes. Combine remaining ingredients and pour into pan. Bake at 375 degrees for 45 minutes. Cool.

Yield: 16 servings   Count: 1 CHO

Apple Cake

1 cup flour

1/2 tsp. each nutmeg and cinnamon

1/4 tsp. salt

3/4 cup sugar

3 Tbsp. margarine, softened

1 egg

2 Tbsp. 1% milk

3 cups baking apples, cored and sliced

Preheat oven to 350 degrees. Spray an 8-inch square pan with nonstick spray. Combine flour through salt and set aside. Beat sugar and margarine together until fluffy; add egg and milk and beat another minute. Add 1/3 of flour mixture at a time and beat until smooth. With a large spoon, stir in apples until evenly distributed. Spread batter in prepared pan. Combine 1 tsp. sugar and 1/2 tsp. cinnamon and sprinkle evenly on the batter. Bake 40 to 45 minutes.

Yield: 12 servings   Count: 1-1/2 CHO

Banana Puff Dessert from Sue Colovos

3	egg whites
1	cup Splenda
12	low-fat saltine crackers, crushed
1	tsp. baking powder
1	tsp. vanilla
2/3	cup walnuts
3	bananas
8	Tbsp. fat-free whipped topping

Beat egg whites until stiff. Fold in sugar and baking powder. Stir in sliced banana and crackers. Spoon into baking dish sprayed with nonstick spray. Bake at 350 degrees for 30 minutes. Serve with fat-free whipped topping.

Yield: 8 servings   Count: 1 CHO

Basic Cake from Cathy Stephens

Cake mix flavor and additions (such as nuts) may be substituted.

1	box spice cake mix
1	can pumpkin
1/2	cup water
1	cup chopped nuts

Spray 13 by 9-inch pan with nonstick spray. Combine all ingredients and bake at 375 degree oven for 45 minutes.

Yield: 24 servings   Count: 1 CHO

Chocolate Almond Meringue Cookies

1/3	cup almonds, ground
1/2	tsp. each cornstarch and cinnamon
1	oz. semisweet chocolate, grated
2	large egg whites at room temperature
1/8	tsp. cream of tartar
3/4	cup powdered sugar
1/4	tsp. almond extract

Preheat oven to 300 degrees. Combine first four ingredients. Beat egg whites and cream of tartar until foamy; gradually add sugar and beat until stiff. Add extract and gently fold in almond mixture. Drop by tablespoons on baking sheet coated with nonstick spray. Bake for 45 minutes; cool on wire rack.

Yield: 2 doz.   Count: 3 cookies = 1 CHO

Chocolate Chip Cookies—milk free---from Michelle Brown

1	cup milk-free margarine (Nucoa or WillowRun)
3/4	cup each brown and white sugar
3	Tbsp. each canola oil and water
2	tsp. baking powder
1	tsp. vanilla
1/4	tsp. salt
2-1/4	cup flour
2	tsp. cornstarch
1/3	cup unsweetened cocoa powder
1	cup milk-free chocolate chips

Beat margarine until fluffy; add sugars. Mix oil, water and baking powder and add to sugar mix; add vanilla. Combine flour, cornstarch, cocoa, baking soda and salt. Blend into mixture. Stir in chips. Drop from spoon onto baking sheet coated with nonstick spray. Bake at 375 degrees for 9 to 11 minutes.

Yield: 3 dozen   Count: 1 cookie = 1 CHO

Chocolate Cookies

8	oz. semi-sweet baking chocolate
3/4	cup brown sugar
1/4	cup margarine
2	eggs
1	tsp. vanilla
1/2	cup flour
1/4	tsp. baking powder

Coarsely chop half the chocolate; melt remaining chocolate in microwave bowl for 1 to 2 minutes; stir until melted and smooth. Stir in sugar, margarine, eggs, and vanilla; then stir in flour and baking powder. Add reserved chocolate chunks. Drop by spoonfuls onto ungreased cookie sheet. Bake 12 minutes at 350 degrees. Cool on wire rack.

Yield: 18 cookies   Count: 1 cookie = 1 CHO

Chocolate Chip Meringue Cookies

3   large egg whites
1/4   tsp. each cream of tartar and salt
1   cup sugar
3   Tbsp. cocoa powder
3   Tbsp. mini chocolate chips

Preheat oven to 300 degrees. Beat egg whites, cream of tartar, and salt until soft peaks form; add sugar 1 Tbsp. at a time, and beat until stiff peaks form. Fold in cocoa powder, then chips. Cover baking sheet with baking parchment. Drop batter by tablespoons onto sheet. Bake for 40 minutes or until crisp. Cool on wire rack.

Yield: 4 dozen   Count: 3 cookies = 1 CHO

Chocolate Mousse from Alexis Scheureman

3/4	cup semi-sweet chocolate chips, melted
1	12.3 oz. pkg. reduced fat extra-firm tofu
1/4	tsp. salt
3	large egg whites
1/2	cup Splenda
1/4	cup water
	Fat free whipped topping (optional)

Place tofu and chocolate in blender and process until smooth. Place salt and egg whites in medium bowl, beat on high until stiff peaks form. Combine Splenda and water in saucepan; bring to boil. Boil for 1 minute. Pour hot syrup in thin stream over egg whites, beating at high speed. Gently stir 1/4 of meringue into the tofu mixture; fold in remaining meringue. Spoon 1/2 cup mousse into each custard cup. Cover and chill for at least 4 hours. Garnish with whipped topping if desired.

Yield: 8 servings   Count: 1/2 CHO 1/2 PRO

Citrus Granita

1-1/4	cup water
1/3	cup sugar
1/4	cup lemon juice
1/4	cup orange juice

Combine ingredients in saucepan. Bring to boil and cook over medium heat for 1 minute or until sugar dissolves, stirring constantly. Remove from heat; cool. Pour into 13 by 9 inch baking dish; cover and freeze until firm.

To serve, scrape entire mixture with tines of fork until fluffy. Cover and freeze for up to a month.

Yield: 5 servings   Count: 1 CHO

Fat-Free and Milk-Free Ice Cream from Karen Kamilos

4	cups Mocha Mix Fat Free
4	bananas
1	tsp. vanilla extract
1	tsp. banana extract
5	tsp. Equal or sugar substitute of choice

Combine all ingredients and freeze according to manufacturer directions; alternate fruits and extracts may be used in place of banana.

Yield: 16 servings of 1/2 cup   Count: 1/2 CHO

Honey Almond Cookie

2	cup flour
1/2	tsp. baking soda
1/8	tsp. salt
1/3	cup sugar
1/3	cup honey
1/4	cup margarine, softened
2	Tbsp. canola oil
1-1/2	tsp. vanilla
1	tsp. almond extract
1	large egg white
1/4	cup sliced almonds, chopped

Combine flour, soda and salt in mixing bowl. Add sugar, honey, margarine, and oil, and beat until well blended. Add egg white and extracts. Dough will be sticky. Coat hands with nonstick spray and divide dough into two portions. Shape into 9″ logs; wrap in plastic wrap; freeze until firm. Preheat oven to 375 degrees. Cut each log into twenty- four slices and place on baking sheet (sprayed with nonstick). Press chopped almonds on top. Bake for 9 minutes. Cool on wire rack.

Yield: 4 dozen   Count: 2 cookies = 1 CHO

Lemon Cookies

2	cups flour
1/4	tsp. each baking powder and salt
2	lemons
3/4	cup butter or margarine
1/2	cup each granulated and powdered sugar
1/2	tsp. vanilla

Blend butter and sugars until creamy; add vanilla, lemon peel, and juice. Add dry ingredients. Divide dough in half and shape into 6 inch log; wrap in waxed paper and chill overnight. To bake slice into 1/4 inch slices; place on ungreased baking sheet. Sprinkle lightly with granulated sugar.

Bake at 350 degrees for 10 minutes or until lightly browned. Cool on wire rack.

Yield: 5 dozen   Count: 3 cookies = 1 CHO

Lemon Cornmeal Cookies

1	cup sugar
3/4	cup butter
2	large eggs
1	Tbsp. grated lemon peel
2	tsp. vanilla
1-1/2	cups each flour and yellow cornmeal
3/4	tsp. baking powder
1/2	tsp. salt

Beat sugar with butter until creamy. At low speed beat in eggs, lemon peel and vanilla. Gradually add remaining ingredients. Divide dough into half and shape into rolls; wrap in plastic wrap and refrigerate overnight. To bake heat oven to 350 degrees. Slice dough into 1/4-inch slices and bake on greased cookie sheet for 15 minutes or until edges are browned. Cool on wire rack.

Yield: 4-1/2 dozen cookies   Count 2 cookies = 1 CHO

Lemon Mousse from Geri Richards

1	lemon, thinly sliced
1	Tbsp. agar flakes
2	cup sugar-free lemonade
3	Tbsp. honey
1	10.5 oz. box firm tofu
6	strawberries for garnish

Combine agar with 1/4 cup lemonade; stir until dissolved. Boil remaining lemonade with lemon slices; reduce heat and simmer for 10 minutes, stirring constantly. Add honey and agar mix; cool. In food processor pulse lemon mix until coarsely chopped. Add tofu in two batches and process until smooth. Divide into six serving dishes; garnish with sliced strawberry.

Yield: 6 servings   Count: 1 CHO 1 PRO

Lime Angel Squares from Cheri DiDio

3   oz. pkg. sugar-free lime gelatin
1   cup boiling water
8˝   prepared angel-food cake, cut into cubes
8   oz. reduced fat (soy) cream cheese, cubed
1/2   cup Splenda
2   tsp. lime juice
1-1/2 tsp. grated lime rind
8   oz. reduced-fat whipped topping, divided

Dissolve gelatin in boiling water. Refrigerate 30 minutes. Place cake cubes in 13 by 9 by 2 inch dish coated with nonstick spray; set aside. Beat cream cheese until smooth. Beat in Splenda, juice and rind. Add gelatin mix; beat until combined. Fold in 1-1/2 cups topping; Spread over cake. Refrigerate 2 hours or until firm. Cut into squares and top each piece with whipped topping.

Yield: 15 servings   Count: 1 CHO

Mango Pudding from Marilyn Gibson

1-1/2 cups boiling water
1/2   cup Splenda
3   pkt. Knox unflavored gelatin
1-1/2 cup cold water
2   mangos
1-1/3 box Mori Nu reduced fat tofu

Dissolve Splenda and gelatin in boiling water. Blend mangos and tofu until smooth; add to gelatin mixture; chill until firm.

Yield: 4 servings   Count: 1 CHO 1 PRO

Mimosa Granita

1   cup water
1   cup sugar
3   cups fresh orange juice (about 10 oranges)
2   cups champagne or sparkling wine
2   Tbsp. fresh lime juice

Combine sugar and water in saucepan; bring to boil, stirring until sugar dissolves. Remove from heat and cool completely. Add remaining ingredients; pour into 11 by 7-inch baking dish. Cover and freeze for 8 hours or until firm. Remove from freezer and let stand for 10 minutes Scrape the entire mixture with a fork until fluffy.

Yield: 8 servings   Count: 1 CHO

Mocha Crumb Cake

1-1/4	cup flour
2/3	cup sugar
3	Tbsp. cocoa powder
1	Tbsp. instant coffee
1/8	tsp. salt
1/4	cup margarine
1/2	tsp. baking powder
1/4	tsp. baking soda
1/3	cup 1% milk (or soy)
1	tsp. vanilla
1	egg

Preheat oven to 350 degrees. Spray 8˝ pan with nonstick spray. Combine flour through salt in mixing bowl. Add margarine and cut in with pastry blender until coarse. Set aside 1/2 cup for topping. Add baking powder and soda, milk, vanilla, and egg. Beat until blended. Spoon into baking pan. Add 1-1/2 tsp water to reserved flour mix and stir with fork. Sprinkle crumb mix over batter. Bake at 350 degrees for 30 minutes. Cut into wedges to serve.

Yield: 16 servings   Count: 1 CHO

Peach Custard Pie from Harry Wrigley

1	single-crust pie shell
1	large egg plus 1 egg white
1	Tbsp. margarine, melted
2	Tbsp. flour or arrowroot, divided plus 1 Tbsp cornstarch
1/4	tsp. almond extract
1/4	cup nonfat half n half or Mocha Mix
1/2	cup plus 2 Tbsp Splenda
2	lb. fresh peaches, sliced

Line shell with foil; shiny side up. Fill with dried beans; bake 10 minutes at 425 degrees. Remove foil and beans; bake 10 minutes longer. Beat egg white with 2 tsp. water; brush shell with this mixture immediately and set aside. Combine peaches, 1 Tbsp. flour and 2 Tbsp. Splenda. Place in crust. Combine remaining ingredients and pour over peaches. Bake 10 minutes at 425 degrees; turn oven down to 350 degrees and bake 40 minutes or until set.

Yield: 16 servings   Count: 1 CHO

Peach Tart from Mary Reese

1	cup water
1	cup Splenda
1	tsp. lemon juice
4	large peaches, cut in half with pit removed
1/2	cup flour
1/8	tsp. salt
3	Tbsp. butter or margarine
	Ice water
1	cup soy milk
1	egg
1/3	cup Splenda
1/4	cup flour
	Pinch salt
1	tsp. vanilla

Combine first three ingredients to make a simple syrup (bring to boil); add peach halves and cook just until beginning to soften. Cool. Remove skin and slice. Combine flour and salt; cut in butter; add ice water and stir just until moistened. Roll thin, and line tart or pie pan with crust. Put sliced peaches on top of crust. Combine remaining ingredients and pour over peaches. Bake at 375 degrees for 35 minutes.

Yield: 10 servings   Count: 1 CHO

Peanut Butter Cookies from Mary and Tom Rupp

1   cup creamy peanut butter
1   cup Splenda
1/4   cup egg substitute
1   tsp. vanilla

Combine all ingredients and roll into 20 balls. Place on ungreased baking sheet and flatten with tines of fork. Bake at 375 degrees for 10 to 12 minutes.

Yield: 20 cookies   Count: 1/2 PRO 1 FAT

Peppermint Mousse Pudding

3   oz. York Peppermint Patties
1/4   cup nonfat milk
1   Tbsp. cocoa powder
1   8 oz. container frozen whipped topping, thawed (do not substitute)
3   drops green or red food color

Remove wrappers from candy and cut into pieces. Place candy, milk, and cocoa in microwave safe bowl. Heat on high for 30 seconds; stir. Repeat as needed until candy is melted and smooth when stirred. Cool slightly. Fold whipped topping into melted mixture and spoon into dessert dishes. Cover and freeze for 3 to 4 hours or until firm. May be garnished with additional whipped topping.

Yield: 8 servings   Count: 1 CHO 1 FAT

Pumpkin Cheesecake

12	gingersnaps, crushed
1	Tbsp. margarine, melted
1	cup 1% cottage cheese
8	oz. light cream cheese
8	oz. fat-free cream cheese
1-1/4	cup sugar
1/2	cup low fat sour cream
2	Tbsp. cornstarch
2	tsp. flour
1	tsp. vanilla
1	tsp. pumpkin pie spice
1	15 oz. can pumpkin
4	large egg whites
2	large eggs

Heat oven to 375 degrees. Spray 9″ spring-form pan with nonstick spray. Combine crumbs and margarine and press into bottom of pan; bake for 5 minutes. Reduce heat to 325 degrees. In food processor, blend cottage cheese until smooth. Add remaining ingredients and mix until smooth. Pour into pan and bake for 1-1/2 hours. Remove from oven and run knife around edge. Cool.

Yield: 24 servings   Count: 1 PRO 1 CHO

Pumpkin Custard from Marge Derdowski

5	egg whites
1	whole egg
1-1/2	cups Mocha Mix Lite
2	tsp. pumpkin pie spice
1/2	cup brown sugar substitute
32	oz. can pumpkin

Combine all ingredients and pour into 11 by 7-inch pan sprayed with nonstick spray. Place custard in larger pan half-filled with water. Bake at 350 degrees for 30 to 40 minutes.

Yield: 6 servings   Count: 1 PRO 1 CHO

Pumpkin Pie from Linda Herzog

1	qt. Breyers Carb Smart Vanilla ice cream
1/2	can pumpkin with spices
1/4	cup crushed Sugar-free Almond Roca
1/2	cup graham cracker crumbs
2	Tbsp. butter, melted

Combine crumbs with butter and press into bottom of pie pan. Mix remaining ingredients and pour into graham cracker crust. Chill for several hours in the freezer. Top with whipped cream sweetened with Splenda.

Yield: 8 servings   Count: 1 CHO

Reduced Fat Fudge

1-1/2 cups Hershey's reduced fat semi-sweet baking chips
2/3   cup low-fat sweetened condensed milk
        Dash salt
3/4   tsp. vanilla extract

Line 9 by 5 by 3 loaf pan with foil. Combine all ingredients in bowl; microwave for 1 minute and stir until chips are melted. Spread into pan. Refrigerate for 2 hours. Remove from pan and remove foil. Cut into 18 pieces.

Yield: 18 pieces   Count: 1 piece = 1 CHO

Strawberry Bavarian from Theda Silcock

1/2	bag whole frozen unsweetened strawberries
1/4	cup low-sugar strawberry preserves
1/4	cup granular sucralose (Splenda)
2	Tbsp. balsamic vinegar
3/4	cup water, divided
2	envelopes, unflavored gelatin
1	Tbsp. honey
1/2	cup pasteurized egg whites
1/2	tsp. cream of tartar
1	tsp. vanilla
1	pt. strawberries, washed and hulled
1	cup light whipped topping, defrosted

Blend frozen strawberries, preserves and sucralose until smooth. Set aside. Combine vinegar with 1/4 cup water in small saucepan; add gelatin and soften. Add remaining 1/2 cup water and honey. Cook over medium heat until gelatin dissolves. Whisk gelatin mixture into berry mix. Refrigerate until thickened, but not set.

Combine egg whites and cream of tartar. Beat until tripled in volume and soft peaks form. Gently fold egg whites, 1/3 at a time, into chilled berry mixture. Pour into pre-chilled 2-quart mold. Refrigerate for 8 hours or overnight.

To serve, run tip of knife around top of mold. Dip mold briefly into large bowl of hot water to loosen. Center a large serving plate on top of the mold. Shake gently to release. Remove mold and refrigerate. To serve you may garnish with whole fresh berries and 2 Tbsp. whipped topping.

Yield: 10 servings   Count: 1 CHO

Sugar Free Cake from Helen Maxwell

2	cups raisins
2	cups water
2	cups whole wheat or white flour
1	tsp. baking soda
1-1/4	tsp. cinnamon
1/2	tsp. nutmeg
1	cup unsweetened applesauce
2	eggs
3/4	cup canola oil
3	pkg. sugar substitute
1/2	cup walnuts, chopped

Cook raisins in water on low heat; stir; cook until liquid is absorbed. Cool. Mix flour, soda, spices and raisins. Add remaining ingredients. Pour into angel food cake pan. Bake at 350 degrees for 30 minutes.

Yield: 30 servings   Count: 1 CHO

Sugar Free Cookies from Helen Maxwell

1	cup raisins
1	cup water
1/4	cup chopped apple
1/2	cup dates
1/2	cup light margarine
1	cup whole wheat or white flour
1	tsp. each baking soda and vanilla
1	cup rolled oats
2	eggs
1	cup chopped walnuts

Boil raisins in water with apples and dates for 3 minutes. Add margarine and cool. Add remaining ingredients. Refrigerate overnight. To bake, heat oven to 350 degrees. Drop by spoonfuls onto ungreased baking sheet. Bake for 10 to 12 minutes.

Yield: 2 dozen   Count: 1 CHO

Sweet Potato Cheesecake from Colleen Perry (milk-free)

2	cups vanilla wafer crumbs (1/2 lb. crushed)
1/2	cup Nucoa margarine, melted
24	oz. Tofutti Better 'n Cream Cheese
1	cup Splenda
1/2	cup light brown sugar
3	eggs, lightly beaten
2	cups cooked mashed sweet potato
1/4	cup Vanilla Silk Milk

1   Tbsp. Vanilla, divided

1   tsp. cinnamon

1-1/2 tsp. nutmeg

1   tsp. lemon juice

2   cup Tofutti Sour Cream

Coat 9 to10″ spring-form pan with margarine and lightly flour. Combine cookie crumbs and melted margarine; press mixture on bottom and up sides of pan. Bake 350 degrees for 12 minutes. Cool. Reduce heat to 325 degrees.

Beat cream cheese until smooth; add 3/4 cup Splenda, brown sugar and eggs. In a separate bowl, combine potato, Silk milk, 1 tsp. vanilla, cinnamon, nutmeg and lemon juice. Add sweet potato mixture to cheese and blend well. Wrap foil around bottom and sides of pan. Pour batter into pan and set in larger pan. Place in middle of oven and pour 1 inch hot water into larger pan. Bake for about 70 minutes or until edges are firm and center is still slightly shaky.

Combine sour cream with remaining Splenda and 2 tsp. vanilla. Remove cheesecake from water bath and pour sour cream topping on top, spreading evenly. Continue baking for 10 minutes. Remove from oven and place on rack to cool for 1 hour. Remove foil and refrigerate for 4 hours or overnight.

Yield: 24 servings   Count: 1 CHO 3 FAT

Tiramisu

12	oz. cream cheese, softened
1	Tbsp. sugar
2	Tbsp. Splenda
1/4	cup brewed coffee, cold
1/2	tsp. vanilla
1	cup frozen light whipped topping
	Additional topping for garnish

Combine first five ingredients and mix until well-blended; refrigerate for 2 hours. Fold in whipped topping. Spoon into dessert dishes. Top with dollop of whipped topping and sprinkle with cocoa powder.

Yield: 8 servings   Count: 3 FAT

Tofu Cheesecake from Mary Reese

15	graham cracker squares
2	Tbsp. sugar
3	Tbsp. Nucoa margarine
19	oz. tofu cream cheese
1	cup sugar
2	tsp. lemon peel
1/4	tsp. vanilla
1	Tbsp. flour
3	eggs

Combine crumbs, 2 Tbsp sugar and margarine and press into 9″ spring-form pan. Bake 300 degrees for 10 minutes. Cool.

Beat cream cheese; add sugar gradually; add peel and vanilla. Beat in eggs one at a time. Bake with a pan of water in the oven in addition to the cheesecake for 1 hour at 350 degrees. Open the door for a few minutes before removing.

For pineapple topping: drain 14 oz. can crushed pineapple in own juice, reserving juice. To the juice add 1 tsp. lemon juice, 2 Tbsp. Splenda, 1 Tbsp. cornstarch; cook until thick and clear; add back drained pineapple; cool, then spread on cheesecake.

Yield: 24 servings   Count: 1 CHO 2 FAT

Tofu Pumpkin Custard

1	16 oz. can pumpkin
1	lb. tofu
1/2	tsp. each allspice and ginger
1	tsp. cinnamon
2	Tbsp. canola oil
1	tsp. vanilla
2/3	cup light brown sugar
1/4	tsp. salt

Combine all ingredients in food processor and process until smooth. Pour into 9-inch pie pan coated with non-stick cooking spray. Bake at 350 degrees for 30 to 35 minutes or until knife inserted in center comes out clean.

Yield: 8 servings   Count: 1/2 PRO 1 CHO

Tofu Pumpkin Pie

1	single-crust pie crust
1	cup reduced fat soft tofu
1-1/2	cup cooked pumpkin
1/2	cup sugar
2	Tbsp. cornstarch
1/2	cup 1% or soy milk
1	egg
2	tsp. pumpkin pie spice

Preheat oven to 400 degrees. Bake pie shell for 5-7 minutes; remove and cool. Reduce heat to 350 degrees. Combine remaining ingredients and pour into shell. Bake for 1 hour. Cool.

Yield: 10 servings   Count: 1 CHO 1/2 PRO

Tofu Whip

1	box Mori Nu reduced fat tofu
2	pkt. Splenda
2	Tbsp. instant sugar-free vanilla pudding mix
2/3	cup soy milk

Blend all ingredients until thick, smooth and creamy. May be combined with a variety of fruits or you can substitute chocolate for the vanilla pudding mix.

Yield: 6 servings   Count: 1/2 PRO

Miscellaneous

Apricot Fruit Snacks

3   cup chopped dried apricots
1/2   cup sugar
1/4   cup water

Combine ingredients in saucepan; bring to boil. Cover and cook 5 minutes or until apricots are tender and sugar dissolves. Blend mixture in food processor until smooth. Pour puree into 15 by 10 inch pan coated with nonstick spray. Bake in 175 degree oven, with oven door partially open, for 8 hours. Peel off pan and roll up. Store in zip-top bag.

Yield: 8 servings   Count: 1 CHO

Blue Goo

1   3 oz. Berry Blue gelatin mix (sugar-free if available)
1/2   cup boiling water
1-1/2 cup nonfat milk

Add boiling water to gelatin, and stir until completely dissolved, 3 to 5 minutes. Pour into medium mixing bowl and stir in milk. Refrigerate until almost set, about 1 hour. Beat at low speed of mixer until it doubles in volume, 3 to 5 minutes.

Yield: 6 servings   Count: 1 CHO.

If made with sugar-free flavor, count as free.

Cannellini Bean Spread

1	16 oz. can white beans, drained
1/4	cup fresh parsley, chopped
2	Tbsp. Italian bread crumbs
2	Tbsp. grated Parmesan cheese
2	Tbsp. water
1	Tbsp. pesto sauce
1	Tbsp. balsamic vinegar

Mash beans and stir in remaining ingredients. Serve as spread with crackers or with artichokes.

Yield: 8 servings.   Count: 1/2 PRO 1/2 CHO

Fajita Marinade

2	cloves garlic, minced
1/2	tsp. each oregano, cumin and salt
2	Tbsp. each orange juice and vinegar

Combine all ingredients. Marinate desired meat in plastic zip-top bag. Cook meat over medium to high heat; discard remaining marinade.

Yield: amount for 1 lb. meat   Count: FREE

Fresh Berry Jam

4   cups berries

1   cup sugar

2   tsp. lemon juice

Combine berries and sugar in saucepan. Bring to simmer over medium high heat. Reduce heat to medium and simmer for 1 hour or until thick, stirring occasionally. Remove from heat; add lemon juice. Cool. Refrigerate to preserve freshness.

Yield: 2 cups   Count: 1 Tbsp. = 1/2 CHO

Jerky from G. Ruffo

1   lb. beef flank steak or turkey breast, sliced thin

1/2   cup soy sauce

1/4   tsp. garlic powder

         Salt to taste

1-2   drops liquid smoke

Marinate sliced meat for 1 to 3 hours. Bake directly on rack in 140 degree oven (place a baking tray or aluminum foil on the rack below to protect from drips) for 8 hours or until dry.

Yield: 10 oz.   Count: 1/2 oz. jerky = 1 PRO

Miniature Meatballs

2	Tbsp. soy sauce
1/4	cup water
1/2	garlic clove, minced
1/2	tsp. nutmeg
1	lb. lean ground beef or turkey

Combine all ingredients and mix lightly. Form into 1-inch balls. Arrange on lightly oiled baking sheet. Bake for 15 minutes at 350 degrees. Place on heated tray and serve with toothpicks.

Yield: 24 meatballs   Count: 1/2 PRO

Navy Bean Spread

1	russet potato, cubed and steamed until tender
2	Tbsp. olive oil
2	cup onion, chopped
4	Tbsp. garlic, chopped
1	16 oz. can navy beans, rinsed
1	tsp. oregano
1	tsp. thyme
4	Tbsp. nonfat plain yogurt or tofu
	Salt and pepper to taste

Sauté vegetables in oil until tender. Add remaining ingredients. Divide into half and blend. Season as desired. Spread on bread or use as a dip with vegetables.

Yield: 3-1/2 cups   Count: 1 Tbsp. = 1 VEG

56 - 1 Tbsp. servings

Parmesan Eggplant Slices

1/4   cup fat-free mayonnaise
1   eggplant, cut into 24 slices
12   saltines, crushed
1/2   cup fresh Parmesan cheese (use sheep Romano for milk-free)

Combine cracker crumbs and cheese in plastic bag. Spread eggplant slices on both sides with mayonnaise; shake in cracker mix to coat. Place on a baking sheet coated with nonstick spray. Chill 2 hours. Preheat oven to 425 degrees. Bake for 15 minutes; turn slices and bake 5 minutes until crisp.

Yield: 4 servings   Count: 1 CHO

Sarah's Rhubarb Chutney

1   lb. rhubarb
1/2   cup distilled vinegar
2   Tbsp. ginger
1   cup sugar or stevia (or sugar substitute of choice)
1/2   tsp. each cinnamon and cloves
1/4   tsp. orange rind
1/2   cup chopped pecans.

Bring to boil everything but the nuts. Simmer until it reaches the consistency of marmalade. Add nuts. Cool. Serve with roast chicken, pork, etc.

Yield: 8 servings   Count: 1 FAT

Roasted Red Pepper Spread

1	clove garlic, peeled
1	Tbsp. olive oil
1	Tbsp. balsamic vinegar
1	15 oz. can garbanzo beans, drained
1	12 oz. jar roasted red peppers, drain and reserve 1 Tbsp. juice
1/4	tsp. salt and 1 Tbsp. water
1	Tbsp. chopped fresh parsley

Put all ingredients in blender or food processor and puree until mixture is smooth. Serve with crackers or fresh vegetables. Store covered in refrigerator for up to 5 days.

Yield: 18 servings   Count: 1/4 CHO

Fresh Salsa

3	large tomatoes, peeled and diced
1/2	cup white onion, chopped fine
1/2	jalapeno pepper, chopped
1	Anaheim pepper, seeded and chopped
1/2	sweet red pepper, chopped
2	Tbsp. cilantro, chopped
1/4	tsp. salt
	Juice from 1/2 lime
1	tsp. white wine vinegar
1	Tbsp. water

Combine all ingredients; let stand for 30 minutes.

Yield: 2 to 3 cups   Count: FREE

Salt-free Herb Rub

2   Tbsp. dried rosemary
2   Tbsp. dried thyme
1   Tbsp. dried tarragon
1   Tbsp. black pepper

Crush all ingredients together. Store in tightly covered container. Use 2 tsp. per pound of beef or pork; 1 tsp. per pound of fish or chicken.

Yield: 1/3 cup   Count: FREE

Protein Shake Ideas

Chocolate Almond

1/4 cup ea. nonfat frozen vanilla yogurt and nonfat milk
1 tsp. cocoa powder
1/4 tsp. almond extract
2 scoops soy or other protein powder (21 g protein)

Pumpkin

1/4 cup canned pumpkin
1/2 tsp. cinnamon
1/8 tsp. nutmeg
3/4 cup nonfat or soy milk
2 scoops soy or other protein powder (21 g protein)

Tropical

1 Tbsp. unsweetened pineapple
2 Tbsp. orange juice
1/4 banana
1/2 cup orange-pineapple Crystal Light
4 ice cubes
2 scoops soy or other protein powder (21 g protein)

Yield: 1 serving each recipe   Count: 3 PRO 1 CHO

Snack Mix

3	cups bran Chex cereal
1-1/2	cups small pretzels
1/2	cup roasted soy nuts
1/4	cup soybean butter
2	Tbsp. honey
1	cup raisins

Heat oven to 250 degrees. Combine cereal, pretzels and soy nuts. Combine soybean butter and honey in small bowl; heat in microwave for 20 to 30 seconds; stir well. Drizzle honey mixture over cereal and stir until coated. Spread mixture in 15 by 10 inch jelly roll pan. Spray with cooking spray. Bake 8 minutes; stir and bake 8 minutes longer. Transfer to sheet of aluminum foil and cool completely. Stir in raisins and serve.

Yield: 8 servings   Count: 1 PRO 3 CHO

Southwest Guacamole

1	large ripe avocado, chunked
1/4	cup low-fat mayonnaise
2	Tbsp. onion, chopped
1/2	tsp. salt
1/4	tsp. pepper
1	jalapeno pepper, seeded and chopped

Mash avocado; stir in remaining ingredients.

Yield: 1 cup or 16 servings   Count: 1 Tbsp. = 1/2 FAT

Spicy Seasoning Rub

2-1/2 Tbsp. paprika
2   Tbsp. garlic powder
1   Tbsp. salt
1   Tbsp. onion powder
1   Tbsp. dried thyme
1   Tbsp. red pepper
1   Tbsp. black pepper
Combine all ingredients and store in airtight container. Add to meat, fish, or poultry prior to cooking.

Yield: 28 servings   Count: FREE

Stir-fry Marinade

2   cloves garlic, minced
1/2   tsp. ground ginger
3   Tbsp. soy sauce
1   Tbsp. cornstarch
1/2   cup broth
Combine all ingredients. Marinate desired meat in plastic zip bag. Cook meat over medium to high heat; discard remaining marinade.

Count: FREE

Strawberry Sauce

2	cups strawberries
3/4	cup orange juice
1/4	cup powdered sugar
2	Tbsp. honey

Combine all ingredients in blender and process until smooth. Serve over ice cream or frozen yogurt.

Yield: 2 cups

Count: 1 Tbsp. = FREE
3 Tbsp. = 1 CHO

Soy Trail Mix

1	cup roasted soy nuts
2	oz. pretzel sticks, broken
1	cup mini shred wheat
1	Tbsp. ranch dip mix

Combine all ingredients in plastic bag.

Yield: 6 servings

Count: 1 PRO 1 CHO

Tofumole

1	12.3 oz. box reduced-fat firm tofu
1	cup chopped seeded tomato
1/4	cup minced green onion
2	Tbsp. bottled salsa
1/2	tsp. chili powder
1/4	tsp. salt and pepper
1	small avocado, peeled and seeded

Blend tofu until smooth. Stir in remaining ingredients. Cover and chill.

Yield: 6 servings   Count: 1/2 PRO 1 FAT

Trail Mix

1/4	cup smooth peanut butter
1/4	cup light maple syrup
2	oz. low fat granola
32	pretzel sticks
1/2	cup raisins
1	cup roasted soy nuts

Preheat oven to 300 degrees. Combine peanut butter and syrup in microwave bowl. Heat for 30 seconds. Combine granola, soy nuts and pretzels. Pour peanut mix over and stir to coat. Spread mix in single layer on pan coated with nonstick spray. Bake for 15 minutes at 300 degrees; stir and bake for 10 minutes more. Remove from oven and cool; add raisins.

Yield: 14 servings   Count: 1 PRO 1 CHO

Whey Protein Bars

1/4	cup corn syrup
1-3/4	cup whey protein isolate
1/3	cup honey
3/4	cup chopped peanuts
1/3	cup peanut butter
2	Tbsp. powdered sugar
1	tsp. vanilla extract
	Melted chocolate

Place corn syrup, honey, peanut butter, and vanilla into mixer; blend for 1 minute. Combine whey, chopped peanuts, and powdered sugar. Add to mixture in mixer; continue to mix until well combined. Press mixture into lightly greased 9″ by 9″ pan. Let sit for 1 hour. Cut into 12 bars. Dip bars into melted chocolate and place on wax paper. Place bars in freezer for 3 to 4 minutes to harden.

Yield: 12   Count: 2 PRO 1 CHO

About the author

Judy Fields, MHS, RD, FADA, is a Registered Dietitian with a Masters Degree in Health systems. She is recognized by her peers as a Fellow in the American Dietetic Association (now the Academy of Nutrition and Dietetics). She is most proud of this designation since there are fewer than 400 of the 72,000 member organization, who have earned this honor. Her career spans 44 years and she has been in private practice for 34 years. She has published numerous articles for professionals and the lay public. In addition she has been honored by the American Heart Association and the American Dietetic Association at the local and national level.

On a personal note, she has maintained a forty pound weight loss for 46 years. This experience has been the basis for creating the E.A.T. Model and the tools for not only losing weight, but keeping it off.

One of her many hobbies includes a hippopotamus collection, in excess of 3000, which has provided the decorative theme for her offices, logo, and illustrations for her presentations.

Index of Charts and Tools

Index of Recipe Categories